A Handbook on
Allergic Rhinitis

A Handbook on
Allergic Rhinitis

Editor-in-Chief

Neeraj Gupta
MBBS DCH DNB (Pediatrics) IDPCCM DAA DPSM FAAAAI
Allergist, Pediatric Intensivist, and Sleep Medicine Specialist
Senior Consultant
Department of Pediatrics
Sir Ganga Ram Hospital
New Delhi, India
A World Allergy Organization designated 'Centre of Excellence'
President, Indian Society of Allergy, Asthma and Sleep (ISAAS)

Section Editors

Narmada Ashok
DNB FIAP FRCPCH DAA PGDDN MBA
Director and Consultant
Pediatrician
Department of Pediatrics
Nalam Medical Center and Hospital
Vellore, Tamil Nadu, India
Fellow, Indian Academy of Pediatrics
Fellow, Royal College of Paediatrics and Child Health

Gayatri S Pandit
MBBS DLO DAA
Consultant ENT Surgeon and
Allergy Specialist
Department of ENT
Samarth ENT and Allergy Centre
Bengaluru
Manipal Hospital
Bengaluru, Karnataka, India

Kasyapi Nagaraju
MS ENT FACI
Director and Senior Consultant
VN Allergy and Asthma
Research Centre
Chennai, Tamil Nadu, India
Faculty in Fellowship and Diploma
Courses of Allergy in India

Rupali Patil Jain
DORL DPAA LLB PGDHHM PGDMLS
ENT Consultant
Allergologist and
Medicolegal Consultant
Director
Arihant Hospital
Warud, Maharashtra, India

Foreword

Krishna Mohan R

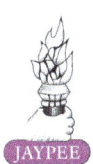

JAYPEE BROTHERS MEDICAL PUBLISHERS
The Health Sciences Publisher
New Delhi | London

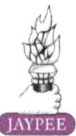 **Jaypee Brothers Medical Publishers (P) Ltd**

Headquarters
Jaypee Brothers Medical Publishers (P) Ltd
EMCA House, 23/23-B
Ansari Road, Daryaganj
New Delhi 110 002, India
Landline: +91-11-23272143, +91-11-23272703
+91-11-23282021, +91-11-23245672
Email: jaypee@jaypeebrothers.com

Corporate Office
Jaypee Brothers Medical Publishers (P) Ltd
4838/24, Ansari Road, Daryaganj
New Delhi 110 002, India
Phone: +91-11-43574357
Fax: +91-11-43574314
Email: jaypee@jaypeebrothers.com

Overseas Office
JP Medical Ltd.
83, Victoria Street, London
SW1H 0HW (UK)
Phone: +44 20 3170 8910
Email: info@jpmedpub.com

EU GPSR Authorised Representative
Logos Europe, 9 rue Nicolas Poussin
17000, La Rochelle, France
Phone: +33 (0) 6 67 93 73 78
E-mail: Contact@logoseurope.eu

Website: www.jaypeebrothers.com
Website: www.jaypeedigital.com

© 2025, Jaypee Brothers Medical Publishers

The views and opinions expressed in this book are solely those of the original contributor(s)/author(s) and do not necessarily represent those of editor(s) or publisher of the book.

All rights reserved. No part of this publication may be reproduced, stored or transmitted in any form or by any means, electronic, mechanical, photocopying, recording or otherwise, without the prior permission in writing of the publishers.

All brand names and product names used in this book are trade names, service marks, trademarks or registered trademarks of their respective owners. The publisher is not associated with any product or vendor mentioned in this book.

Medical knowledge and practice change constantly. This book is designed to provide accurate, authoritative information about the subject matter in question. However, readers are advised to check the most current information available on procedures included and check information from the manufacturer of each product to be administered, to verify the recommended dose, formula, method and duration of administration, adverse effects and contraindications. It is the responsibility of the practitioner to take all appropriate safety precautions. Neither the publisher nor the author(s)/editor(s) assume any liability for any injury and/or damage to persons or property arising from or related to use of material in this book.

This book is sold on the understanding that the publisher is not engaged in providing professional medical services. If such advice or services are required, the services of a competent medical professional should be sought.

Every effort has been made where necessary to contact holders of copyright to obtain permission to reproduce copyright material. If any have been inadvertently overlooked, the publisher will be pleased to make the necessary arrangements at the first opportunity.

Inquiries for bulk sales may be solicited at: jaypee@jaypeebrothers.com

A Handbook on Allergic Rhinitis

First Edition: **2025**

ISBN: 978-93-5696-588-1

Dedicated to

My beloved family, for their unwavering support and boundless patience throughout this journey. Your love and encouragement have been my constant source of strength.

My esteemed mentors and colleagues, whose guidance and insights have profoundly shaped my professional path.

All the patients who have inspired this work with their courage and resilience. This handbook is dedicated to you in hopes of making your journey a bit easier and your days brighter.

Neeraj Gupta

Contributors

Aabid M Koul
MS PhD
Senior Resident
Department of Immunology and
Molecular Medicine
Sher-i-Kashmir Institute of Medical
Sciences
Srinagar, Jammu and Kashmir, India

Amit Suyal
MBBS MD (Pediatrics) DPAA
Consultant and Head
Department of Pediatrics
Krishna Hospital and Research Centre
Haldwani, Uttarakhand, India

Antarbhai Patel
MBBS DCH DNB (Pediatrics) Fellowship PICU
Fellow
Department of Pediatric Pulmonology
and Intensive Care
Sir Ganga Ram Hospital
New Delhi, India

Ayaz Gull
PhD
Senior Research Fellow
Department of Immunology and
Molecular Medicine
Sher-i-Kashmir Institute of Medical
Sciences
Srinagar, Jammu and Kashmir, India

Deepak Kumar
MBBS MD (Pediatrics) Fellowship in Pediatric
Pulmonology and Allergy
Consultant, Pediatric Pulmonologist,
Allergy and Sleep Specialist
Department of Pediatrics
Max Super Speciality Hospital
Sitaram Bhartia Institute of Science and
Research, New Delhi, India

Dinesh Naik
MD MRCPCH DPAA
Specialist Pediatrician
Department of Pediatrics
Al Sharq Hospital
Fujairah, UAE

Gayatri S Pandit
MBBS DLO DAA
Consultant ENT Surgeon and
Allergy Specialist
Department of ENT
Samarth ENT and Allergy Centre
Bengaluru
Manipal Hospital
Bengaluru, Karnataka, India

Gouthami P
MBBS DNB DPAA PGPN
Associate Professor
Pediatric Allergy and
Asthma Specialist
Department of Pediatrics
RVM Institute of Medical Sciences
Hyderabad, Telangana, India

Hima Mathews P
MBBS DCH DNB (Pediatrics) DPAA FAAP
Senior Consultant and Allergist
Department of Pediatrics
Lisie Hospital
Ernakulam, Kerala, India

Kashinath G Metri
BAMS MD PhD
Associate Professor
Department of Yoga
Central University of Rajasthan
Ajmer, Rajasthan, India

Kasyapi Nagaraju
MS ENT FACI
Director and Senior Consultant
VN Allergy and Asthma
Research Centre
Chennai, Tamil Nadu, India
Faculty in Fellowship and Diploma
Courses of Allergy in India

Muzima Jeelani
MSc
MSc Intern
University of Kashmir
Srinagar, Jammu and Kashmir, India

Narmada Ashok
DNB FIAP FRCPCH DAA PGDDN MBA
Director and Consultant
Pediatrician
Department of Pediatrics
Nalam Medical Center and Hospital
Vellore, Tamil Nadu, India
Fellow, Indian Academy of Pediatrics
Fellow, Royal College of Paediatrics and
Child Health

R Prasanna
DCH DNB MRCPCH (UK) MRCP (Edinburgh)
DPAA
Professor
Department of Pediatrics and
Neonatology
SRM Medical College Hospital and
Research Centre
Chengalpattu, Tamil Nadu, India

Roohi Rasool
MBBS MD
Professor
Department of Immunology and
Molecular Medicine
Sher-i-Kashmir Institute of Medical
Sciences
Srinagar, Jammu and Kashmir, India

Rupali Patil Jain
DORL DPAA LLB PGDHHM PGDMLS
ENT Consultant
Allergologist and
Medicolegal Consultant
Director
Arihant Hospital
Warud, Maharashtra, India

Samyugtha R
MBBS DNB (Pediatrics) DPAA
Consultant Pediatrician and
Neonatologist
Department of Pediatrics
KR Hospital
Coimbatore, Tamil Nadu, India

Shebna A Khader
MBBS MD (Pediatrics) DPAA
Consultant Pediatrician and
Pediatric Allergist
ALLERGO KIDZ Pediatric Allergy Clinic
Midtown Medical Centre
Kochi, Kerala, India

Soundarya M
MD (Pediatrics) ACME DPAA
Consultant Pediatric Allergist
Department of Pediatrics
Kasturba Medical College Hospitals
Mangalore, Karnataka, India

Swati Kalra
MBBS MD (Pediatrics) DPAA
Senior Consultant
Department of Pediatrics
Medanta—The Medicity
Gurugram, Haryana, India

Swikaar H Panchal
MBBS MD (Pediatrics) IDPCCM DPAA
Clinical Associate, IPCU
Department of Pediatrics
Bai Jerbai Wadia Hospital for Children
Mumbai, Maharashtra, India

Tabasum Shafi
PhD
Senior Research Fellow
Department of Immunology and
Molecular Medicine
Sher-i-Kashmir Institute of Medical
Sciences
Srinagar, Jammu and Kashmir, India

Taha A Qureshi
MBBS PhD DAA DPAA FAAI
Senior Allergologist
Allergist-Allergy Division
Department of Medicine
Government JLNM Hospital
Srinagar, Jammu and Kashmir, India

Veena Singh Gupta
MD (Pediatrics) DPAA
Senior Consultant
Department of Pediatrics
NC Jindal Institute of
Medical Sciences
New Delhi, India

Foreword

In the labyrinth of modern medical challenges, allergic rhinitis stands out as both a common and a complex condition, affecting millions globally. Despite its prevalence, the nuanced understanding and effective management of this ailment often elude many. It is within this context that Neeraj Gupta's *A Handbook on Allergic Rhinitis* emerges as 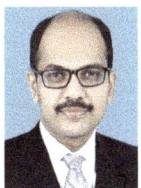 an indispensable resource, bridging the gap between clinical expertise and practical application.

Neeraj Gupta and colleagues, with their extensive experience and profound insight into the realm of allergies, bring forth a comprehensive guide that is both informative and accessible. This handbook is meticulously crafted, reflecting a blend of scientific rigor and empathetic patient care. Author's approach is holistic, considering not only the physiological aspects of allergic rhinitis but also its psychological and social impacts.

The book begins by laying a solid foundation, delving into the epidemiology and pathophysiology of allergic rhinitis. It systematically navigates through diagnostic strategies, ensuring that readers are equipped with the knowledge to identify the condition accurately. The detailed exploration of various treatment modalities, including pharmacological interventions, immunotherapy, and lifestyle modifications, provides a well-rounded perspective essential for effective management.

What sets this handbook apart is its emphasis on personalized care. Neeraj Gupta underscores the importance of tailoring treatment plans to individual patient needs, acknowledging the variability in symptom presentation and response to therapy. This patient-centered approach is further enhanced by practical tips, which enrich the reader's understanding and application of theoretical knowledge.

Moreover, Neeraj Gupta's work is not just a clinical manual but also a beacon of hope for patients and caregivers. By demystifying allergic rhinitis and presenting actionable solutions, the handbook empowers readers to take proactive steps toward managing the condition and improving quality of life.

In an era where information is abundant yet often overwhelming, *A Handbook on Allergic Rhinitis* stands as a beacon of clarity and expertise. It is an essential addition to the library of healthcare professionals, medical students, and anyone seeking a deeper understanding of allergic rhinitis. The team's dedication and scholarly prowess shine through every page, making this handbook a cornerstone reference in the field of allergy and immunology.

As you embark on this journey through the pages of Neeraj Gupta's Handbook, you may find not only knowledge but also inspiration to tackle allergic rhinitis with renewed confidence and compassion.

Krishna Mohan R
Chairperson
IAP Allergy and Applied Immunology Chapter, 2024

Preface

Allergic rhinitis is a condition that touches the lives of countless individuals worldwide, manifesting in symptoms that range from mildly irritating to profoundly disruptive. Despite its common occurrence, the path to effective diagnosis and treatment can often be fraught with complexity and confusion. It is this intricate landscape that *A Handbook on Allergic Rhinitis* seeks to illuminate, providing a clear, comprehensive guide to understanding, and managing this pervasive condition.

My journey into the realm of allergic rhinitis began early in my medical career, spurred by both professional encounters and personal experiences. I have witnessed firsthand the frustration of patients grappling with persistent symptoms, the challenges clinicians face in tailoring effective treatments, and the ongoing evolution of research in this field. These experiences have fueled my commitment to create a resource that demystifies allergic rhinitis and offers practical and evidence-based solutions.

This handbook is designed to serve a diverse audience. For healthcare professionals, it provides an in-depth exploration of epidemiology, pathophysiology, and diagnostic techniques essential for accurate identification and treatment. For medical students and residents, it offers foundational knowledge enhanced by case studies and clinical scenarios to bridge theory and practice. For patients and caregivers, it presents accessible information and actionable advice to navigate the condition with confidence and ease.

The structure of the book is intentional, beginning with a thorough overview of allergic rhinitis, followed by detailed sections on diagnostic strategies and treatment options. Each chapter is crafted to build upon the last, ensuring a cohesive and comprehensive understanding of the subject matter. Emphasis is placed on a patient-centered approach, recognizing the unique presentation of allergic rhinitis in each individual and the necessity of personalized treatment plans.

In writing this handbook, I have drawn upon the latest research, clinical guidelines, and the collective wisdom of my colleagues. I am deeply grateful to the many mentors and peers who have shared their knowledge and insights, contributing to the richness of this work. Special thanks are due to my family, whose unwavering support has been invaluable throughout this endeavor.

I hope that *A Handbook on Allergic Rhinitis* serves as a trusted companion for those seeking to deepen their understanding of this condition and improve the lives of those affected by it. May it inspire confidence, foster empathy, and promote excellence in care.

Thank you for embarking on this journey with me.

Neeraj Gupta

Acknowledgments

The creation of *A Handbook on Allergic Rhinitis* has been a journey marked by collaboration, support, and inspiration from many remarkable individuals and institutions. It is with deep gratitude that I acknowledge those who have contributed to this endeavor.

First and foremost, I extend my heartfelt thanks to my family. Your unwavering support, patience, and encouragement have been the cornerstone of my efforts. To my wife, whose understanding and love have been my constant source of strength, and to my children, who have been a continuous source of joy and motivation, I am profoundly grateful.

I would like to express my sincere appreciation to my mentors and colleagues, whose guidance and expertise have significantly shaped this work. Your insights and constructive feedback have been invaluable. Special thanks to Dr Anil Sachdev, whose mentorship and encouragement have been pivotal in my professional development.

A special note of thanks to the patients who have shared their experiences and stories with me. Your resilience and courage have been a source of inspiration, and it is my hope that this handbook will, in turn, provide you with practical tools and knowledge to better manage allergic rhinitis.

I am deeply grateful to Shri Jitendar P Vij (Group Chairman), Mr Ankit Vij (Managing Director), Mr MS Mani (Group President), Ms Chetna Malhotra (Senior Director—Professional Publishing, Marketing, and Business Development), Ms Pooja Bhandari [Director—Production (Books and Journals)], and Mr Akhilesh Saxena (Publishing Coordinator) of M/s Jaypee Brothers Medical Publishers (P) Ltd, New Delhi, India, for their professional support and dedication to bringing this book to life.

I, along with my team of section editors, would also like to acknowledge the contributions of many researchers and clinicians whose work is cited in this handbook. Your dedication to advancing the understanding and treatment of allergic rhinitis has laid the foundation for this book.

To my friends and colleagues in the medical community, thank you for your encouragement and for fostering an environment of collaboration and continuous learning. Your support has been instrumental in the completion of this project.

Finally, I am grateful to the readers of this handbook. Your quest for knowledge and commitment to improving the management of allergic rhinitis is the ultimate motivation behind this work. It is my hope that this book serves as a valuable resource in your journey.

Thank you all for your support, inspiration, and contributions.

Neeraj Gupta

Contents

SECTION 1: Pathophysiology

Section Editor: S Narmada Ashok

1. **Upper Airway Physiology** 3
   Gouthami P

2. **Rhinitis Classification** 19
   Hima Mathews P

3. **Allergic Rhinitis: Pathophysiology** 32
   Soundarya M

4. **Allergic Rhinitis: Comorbidities** 41
   Swati Kalra

SECTION 2: Diagnostics

Section Editor: Gayatri S Pandit

5. **Clinical Diagnosis: Rhinitis and Comorbidities** 51
   Dinesh Naik

6. **Structural Assessment** 66
   Veena Singh Gupta

7. **Functional Assessment** 79
   Swikaar H Panchal

8. **Inflammatory Assessment in Allergic Rhinitis** 104
   Antarbhai Patel

9. **Allergy Tests** 115
   Taha A Qureshi, Tabasum Shafi, Ayaz Gull,
   Aabid M Koul, Muzima Jeelani, Roohi Rasool

SECTION 3: Therapeutics

Section Editor: Kasyapi Nagaraju

10. **Controllers** 131
    Shebna A Khader

11. **Preventers** 146
    Samyugtha

12. **Disease Modifiers** 158
    R Prasanna

13. **Surgical Intervention in Allergic Rhinitis** 173
    Deepak Kumar

SECTION 4: Prevention, Alternative Medicine, and the Way Ahead

Section Editor: Rupali Patil Jain

14. **Preventive Measures** 183
    Amit Suyal

15. **Evidence-based Complementary and Alternative Medicine for Allergic Rhinitis** 196
    Kashinath G Metri

16. **Futuristic View** 209
    Rupali Patil Jain

Index 221

SECTION 1

Pathophysiology

Section Editor: S Narmada Ashok

- ◈ **Upper Airway Physiology**
  Gouthami P

- ◈ **Rhinitis Classification**
  Hima Mathews P

- ◈ **Allergic Rhinitis: Pathophysiology**
  Soundarya M

- ◈ **Allergic Rhinitis: Comorbidities**
  Swati Kalra

CHAPTER 1

Upper Airway Physiology

Gouthami P

■ INTRODUCTION

Upper airways play a critical role in allergic rhinitis, a highly prevalent, benign, and chronic form of atopy. The disease exceeds >50% of an allergist's office practice with a global burden of 25% and 40% of prevalence in children and adults respectively. Furthermore, the coexistence with other allergic conditions, such as asthma, eczema, and food allergies, increases its overall impact. The symptoms reflect exaggerated defensive and homeostatic functions of the upper airways. Hence, a thorough understanding of the anatomy and physiology of the upper airways is essential for tailoring preventive and treatment strategies.

■ NOSE: ANATOMY

The nose has an external and internal structure, each with distinct features and functions.

Anatomy of External Nose

The nose is externally pyramidal in shape, sloping upward, and posteriorly to reach the forehead at a junction marked by a slight depression called the nasion. The osteocartilaginous framework of the nose is covered by muscles and skin.

Osteocartilaginous framework consists two nasal bones and upper lateral cartilages, lower lateral cartilage is also known as alar cartilages and lesser alar cartilage is also known as sesamoid cartilage and septal cartilage.

The procerus muscle, nasalis with transverse and alar parts, levator labii superioris alaeque nasi, anterior and posterior dilator naris, and depressor septi nasi form the nasal musculature.

The skin on the nasal bones is thin and mobile. The alar cartilages are covered by thick and adherent skin and contain sebaceous glands.

Anatomy of Internal Nose

Nasal septum divides the internal nose into right and left nasal cavities. Each cavity has a naris or nostril to communicate with the exterior. The aperture or the choana forms the communication between nasal cavity and nasopharynx.

The *nasal vestibule* is the most anterior part of the nasal cavity. The area is lined by skin with hair follicles and sebaceous glands. The upper limit on the lateral wall that forms the internal boundary of vestibule is called limen nasi or nasal valve.

Nasal Cavity

Palatine processes of maxillary bones and horizontal process of palatine bone forms the floor of the nasal cavity and cribriform plate constitutes the major portion of the roof of the nasal cavity along with the nasal bones.

Structure of the Lateral Wall

The interior surface of the maxillae, the lacrimal bones, and medial pterygoid make up the lateral wall along with turbinates **(Fig. 1)**.

Turbinates and meatus: Turbinates or the conchae are the scroll-like pitted bones. They are three in number. The inferior turbinate, middle turbinate, and superior turbinate on each side of the nose divide the lumen of nasal cavity into inferior meatus, middle meatus, and superior meatus, respectively.

The *inferior turbinate* is an independent bony projection from the lateral wall of the nose. Inferior meatus is the space beneath the inferior turbinate. The nasolacrimal duct opens laterally in the inferior meatus. The terminal end of the nasolacrimal duct is guarded by a mucosal valve called "Hasner's valve."

The *middle turbinate* develops from the ethmoid bone. Middle meatus lies underneath the turbinate. The middle turbinate is attached in an "S"-shaped

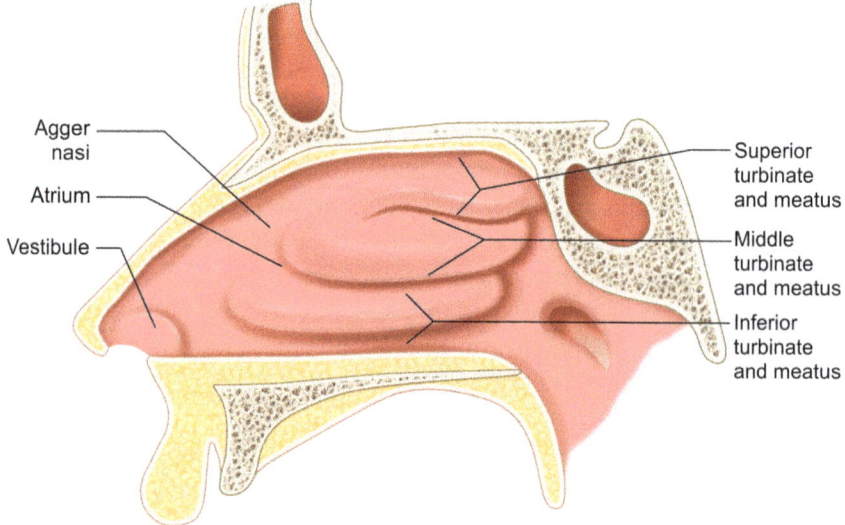

Fig. 1: Lateral wall of the nose.

manner by a bony lamella called the basal lamella. A hook-like structure with a posterosuperior sharp border running parallel to the anterior border of the bulla ethmoidalis is called uncinate process **(Fig. 2)**.

The area limited by the uncinate process, frontal process of maxilla, and sometimes lacrimal bone on the inside, and the lamina papyracea **(Fig. 3)** on the outside is called the "infundibulum." The frontal, maxillary, and anterior ethmoid sinuses drain into the infundibulum.

The sphenoid sinus opens through the sphenoid recess. This opening lies medially on the superior turbinate. The posterior ethmoid cells drain into the central part of the superior meatus.

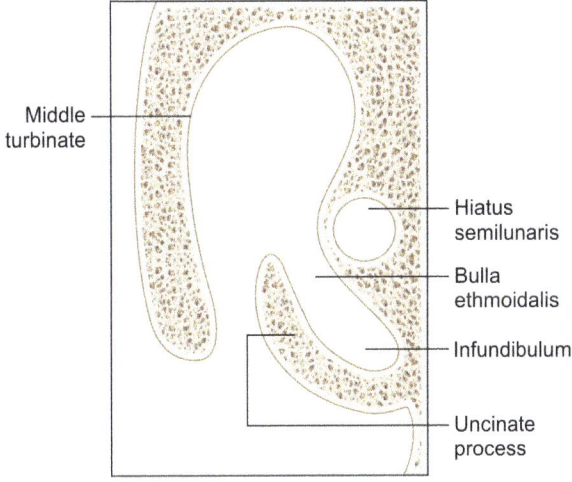

Fig. 2: Coronal section through middle meatus.

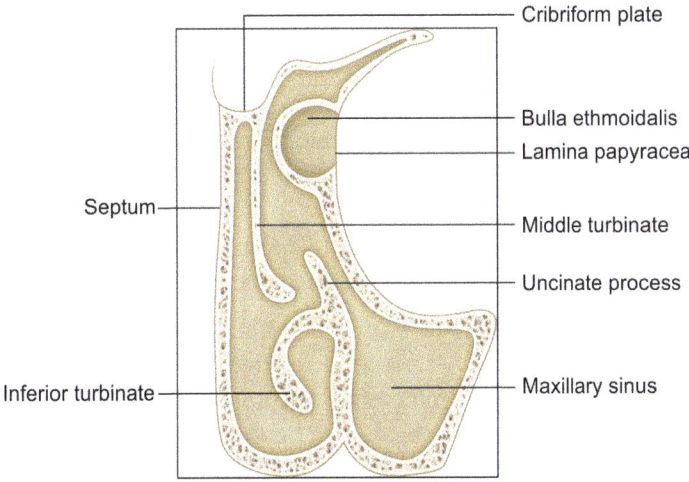

Fig. 3: Ostiomeatal unit.

Nerve supply: The smell sensation is carried by olfactory nerves. Afferent impulses from olfactory nerves are carried to the olfactory region of the cerebral cortex, passing through the cribriform plate. Injury to these nerves can lead to cerebrospinal fluid (CSF) rhinorrhea or meningitis.

Anterior ethmoidal nerve, branches of the sphenopalatine ganglion, and branches of the infraorbital nerve form the innervation of the nasal vestibule.

Autonomic innervation: The function of vasodilation of the blood vessels and secretions from the nasal glands is carried out by parasympathetic nerve fibers from the greater superficial petrosal nerve. The sympathetic nerve fibers originate from the upper two thoracic segments of the spinal cord. Vasoconstriction of the blood vessels in the nose is carried out by these fibers. The nerve of the pterygoid canal also known as vidian nerve is formed by these sympathetic nerves. Sectioning the vidian nerve can control rhinorrhea, a predominant symptom of vasomotor and allergic rhinitis.

Lymphatics from the upper part of the nasal cavity travel along the olfactory nerves to reach the subarachnoid space. The lymphatic drainage of the external nose and anterior part of the nasal cavity is into the submandibular lymph nodes, while the rest of the nasal cavity drains into upper jugular nodes. The blood supply of the nose is predominantly derived from both internal and external carotid artery systems.

■ NOSE: PHYSIOLOGY

Functions

- *Respiration:* Inspiration and expiration
- Conditioning of inspired air (warmth and humidification)
- *Protection of the terminal airways:* Defense mechanisms
- Resonance
- Nasal reflex
- *Olfaction:* Sense of smell

Respiratory mucous membrane: Respiratory area of the nose, trachea, and some parts of the bronchi are lined by pseudostratified ciliated mucosal membrane called "respiratory mucosa." The intercellular spaces are irregularly aligned in this mucosal layer. This facilitates the accommodation of fluid and inflammatory cells, further enhancing the immune response.

Respiration: The air currents during inspiration and expiration passes through the nasal cavities. Air passes through the middle part of the nose during quiet inspiration. Olfactory region is not aerated in quiet breathing. Hence, weak odorous substances need to be sniffed to perceive the sense of smell. During expiration, the air currents are subjected to friction facilitating the ventilation of the sinuses.

Nasal cycle: Rhythmic cyclical congestion and decongestion once in every 2.5–4 hours mediated by parasympathetic and sympathetic innervation of the nose is called "nasal cycle."

Air conditioning: The nose helps to condition the inspired air by heating it and adjusting its humidity. It also filters and purifies the air by trapping dust, pollen, bacteria, and other particulate matter. The countercurrent flow of blood aids in the efficiency of the system.

Protection of lower airways: The ciliary beat and mucous blanket on the nasal mucosa help protect the lower airways. The movement of cilia gets desynchronized by dry air currents, certain drugs, extreme heat or cold, cigarette smoke, vehicle exhaust, viruses, and chemical fumes.

Vocal resonance: The nose forms a resonating chamber for certain consonants (M/N/NG) in speech.

Nasal reflexes: Smell of palatable food can cause reflex secretion of saliva and gastric juice. Irritation of nasal mucosa causes sneezing, and nasal obstruction can lead to increased pulmonary resistance due to tonsil and adenoid hypertrophy.

■ PARANASAL SINUSES: ANATOMY

The mucous membrane of the lateral wall of the nose outpouches into air-filled cavities called "paranasal sinuses." They are divided into two groups **(Table 1)**. The *anterior group* comprises the maxillary, frontal, and anterior ethmoidal sinuses. The openings from these sinuses are directed into the middle meatus **(Fig. 4)**. The *posterior group* comprises the posterior ethmoidal sinuses and sphenoid sinus. Posterior ethmoid sinuses open into the superior meatus, and the sphenoid sinus opens into the sphenoethmoidal

TABLE 1: Paranasal sinuses overview.

	Maxillary	*Ethmoid*	*Frontal*	*Sphenoid*
Embryology	This sinus is the first one to develop. It is formed along the inferolateral surface of the ethmoidal portion of the nasal capsule	Evaginates from lateral nasal wall	An upward extension from frontal recess	Evaginates from the mucosa of sphenoethmoidal recess
Status at birth	Present	Present	Not present	Not present

Contd...

Contd...

	Maxillary	**Ethmoid**	**Frontal**	**Sphenoid**
Growth	Rapid growth occurs from birth to 3 years and a second peak in growth occurs at 7–12 years. Adult size is attained by 15 years of age. Volume is 6–8 mL	Adult size attained by 2 years of age	Complete development occurs by 20 years of age	Full size is attained between 15 years to adult age
Radiological evidence	Appreciated at 4–5 months of age	1 year of age	6 years of age	4 years of age
Blood supply	Maxillary artery. Sinus walls drain into the pterygoid plexus through the maxillary vein	Nasal branches of sphenopalatine artery	Ophthalmic artery supplies the sinus through supratrochlear and suborbital branches	Branches of the sphenopalatine and posterior ethmoid arteries

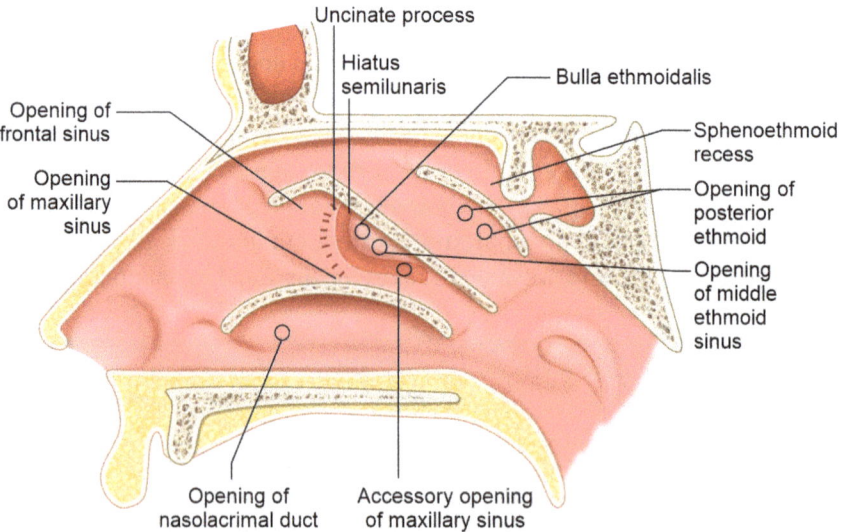

Fig. 4: Opening of various sinuses on the lateral wall of the nose with reflected turbinates.

recess **(Fig. 4)**. There is a thin and ciliated mucous membrane lining the sinuses. The ciliary beat propels the mucous toward the ostia of the sinuses to join the mucous blanket in the nose.

■ PARANASAL SINUSES: PHYSIOLOGY

The air currents traverse the paranasal sinuses through their openings. During breathing in, the sinuses are emptied of air, and during breathing out, they are filled with air.

The sinuses play a physiological role in conditioning the air, voice resonance, acting as thermal insulators and buffers against trauma, protecting vulnerable structures in the orbit and cranium from temperature fluctuations, providing an extended surface for olfaction, and offering local immunological defense against microbes.

■ EAR: ANATOMY

The ear is a vital sense organ responsible for hearing and balance. It consists of three main parts: (1) An external ear, (2) middle ear, and (3) the inner ear **(Fig. 5)**.

The *external anatomy of the ear* includes an external auditory canal, an auricle, and the cartilaginous part of the ear.

The *auricle* comprises helix and antihelix as well as the tragus and antitragus. A scaphoid depression located behind the external auditory meatus is called "concha." It is surrounded by the auricle.

External Auditory Canal

The cartilaginous extension of the auricle forms the outer half of the external auditory canal. The mastoid and tympanic portion of the temporal bone

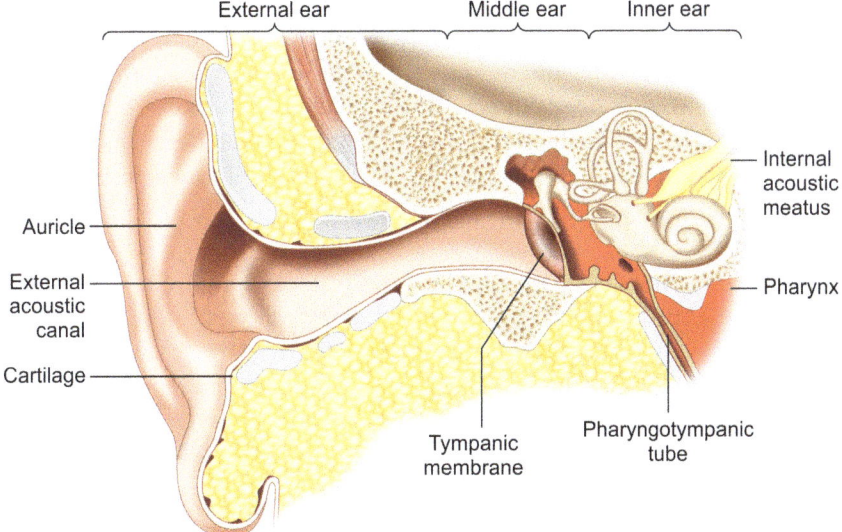

Fig. 5: Ear and its divisions.

forms the inner half of the canal. The canal is limited internally by the tympanic membrane. The skin in the bony part of the canal is taut with minimal subcutaneous tissue underneath. There are numerous hair follicles, ceruminous glands, and sebaceous glands in the region.

The tympanic membrane is also known as eardrum. It is an obliquely set partition between the external acoustic canal and the middle ear. The membrane comprises three layers.

Outer Layer

This layer is continuous with the lining of the external acoustic meatus (ear canal).

Middle Fibrous Layer

This layer provides structural support to the tympanic membrane and helps to maintain the shape and integrity.

Inner Mucosal Layer

This layer is continuous with the mucous lining of the middle ear cavity, keeping the tympanic membrane moist. The tympanic membrane is divided into a lax portion called "pars flaccida" and a taut portion called "pars tensa." A small depressed area known as umbo corresponds to the attachment point of the handle of the malleus.

A small, air-filled cavity located in the temporal bone of the skull, between the tympanic membrane (eardrum) and the inner ear forms the *middle ear cavity* (**Fig. 6**). Three small bones, (1) the malleus (hammer), (2) incus (anvil), and (3) stapes (stirrup), form a chain that runs through the middle ear cavity. They connect the tympanic membrane to the oval window of the inner ear. The oval window is a membrane-covered opening located at the entrance to the inner ear and is connected to the stapes bone of the middle ear. The round window is another opening. A membrane covers this opening. The round membrane serves as a pressure-relief mechanism.

Eustachian Tube

The tubular connection between the nasopharynx and the middle ear is known as the eustachian tube. This connection is responsible for maintaining the balance of pressures between the middle ear and the atmosphere. The tensor tympani and stapedius are the muscles in the middle ear. The physiological role of these muscles is to dampen loud noises.

Inner Ear

Inner ear is located within the temporal bone of the skull. The inner ear cavity consists of a spiral-shaped and fluid-filled structure known as the

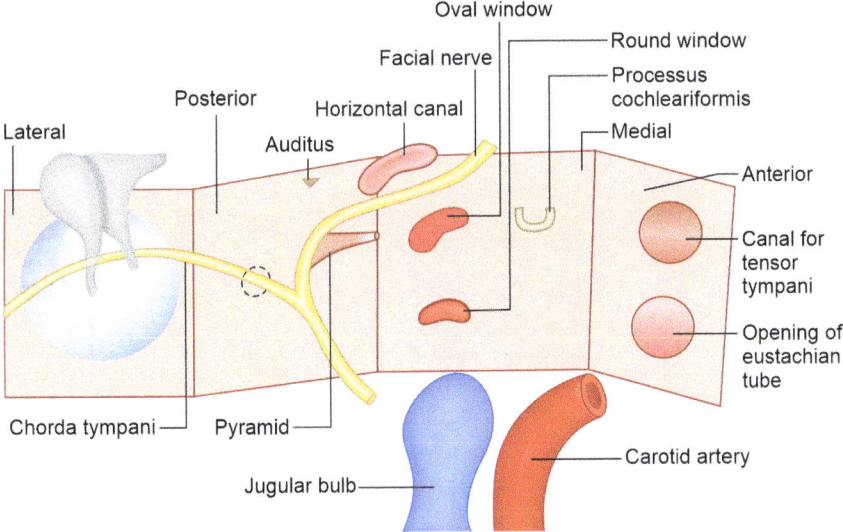

Fig. 6: Structures of middle ear and their relations.

cochlea. There are three fluid-filled chambers: (1) The scala vestibuli, (2) the scala media (cochlear duct), and (3) the scala tympani. Scala media have specialized sensory cells called hair cells forming the organ of Corti. These hair cells convert mechanical vibrations into electrical signals. The auditory nerve transmits these signals to the brain.

Vestibular System

The three semicircular canals constitute the vestibular system. They are responsible for balance, spatial orientation, and coordination of movements. The utricle and saccule, along with sensory hair cells, are two otolith organs located within the vestibule of the inner ear that detect linear acceleration, head position, and changes in gravitational forces.

■ EAR: PHYSIOLOGY

The ear is involved in complex processes related to hearing and balance **(Flowchart 1)**.

Balance physiology: Linear acceleration and head position relative to gravity are maintained by the three semicircular canals, utricle, and saccule. Signals from the vestibular system are transmitted through the vestibular nerve to the brain stem to adjust tone and posture. Dysfunction in any part of the auditory or vestibular system can lead to hearing loss, dizziness, vertigo, and other balance disorders.

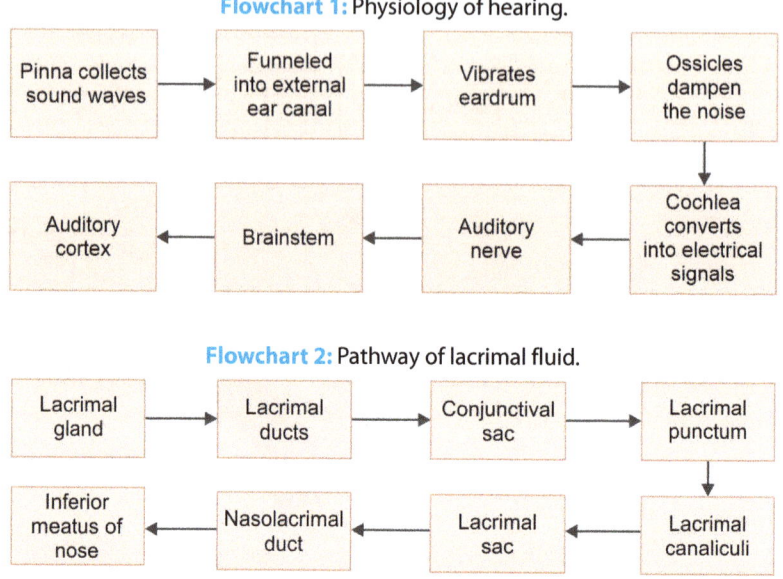

Flowchart 1: Physiology of hearing.

Flowchart 2: Pathway of lacrimal fluid.

Valsalva maneuver: Exposure to changes in altitude causes disturbances of pressure in the middle ear. Valsalva maneuver is an adaptive mechanism that is carried out by forceful exhalation against a closed airway (such as by pinching the nose closed and attempting to blow air out) to balance the pressure in the middle ear. This is facilitated by opening of the eustachian tube, allowing airflow into the middle ear.

■ LACRIMAL APPARATUS

The superolateral aspect of the orbit in the lacrimal fossa accommodates a compound tubuloacinar gland labeled as lacrimal gland. The gland has an orbital part and a palpebral part. The lacrimal apparatus is responsible for draining lacrimal fluid from the orbit **(Flowchart 2)**.

The lacrimal gland is innervated by a branch of the ophthalmic nerve known as the lacrimal nerve. Additionally, it receives parasympathetic innervation from the greater petrosal nerve, which stimulates fluid secretion. The sympathetic innervation of the gland develops from the superior cervical ganglion, which inhibits fluid secretion.

■ PHARYNX

A conical fibromuscular tube of 12–14 cm long, extending from the base of the skull to the lower border of the cricoid cartilage is called "pharynx." The pharynx forms a connection with the esophagus at the level of cricoid cartilage. The width of the base of the pharynx is 3.5 cm and the width at the pharyngoesophageal junction is 1.5 cm. The pharyngoesophageal junction is the narrowest part of the digestive tract.

Pharynx is anatomically divided into three regions **(Fig. 7)**:
1. The nasopharynx or epipharynx
2. The oropharynx
3. The hypopharynx or laryngopharynx

Nasopharynx or Epipharynx

The uppermost part of the throat, behind the nasal cavities, is called "nasopharynx." The structure develops from the base of the skull extending to the soft palate. This level is marked by the horizontal plane passing through the hard palate.

Nasopharyngeal tonsil (adenoids): Pyramid-shaped collections of lymphoid tissue in the nasopharynx are termed as adenoids. They are composed of respiratory epithelium with interspersed seromucous glands. They contribute to immune defense by aiding in the development of T lymphocytes and B lymphocytes. M cells are the specialized cells developed to capture pathogens. This role is carried out by activating B lymphocytes to produce immunoglobulin A (IgA) and establish immunologic memory. Adenoid enlargement blocks breathing resulting in snoring, obstructive sleep apnea, and comorbidities such as serous otitis and sinusitis. Adenoid hypertrophy

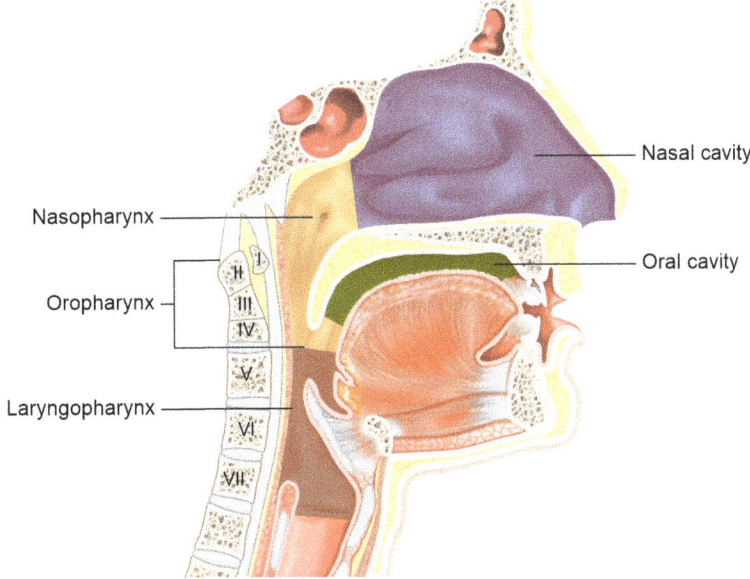

Fig. 7: Anatomical divisions of pharynx and the vertebrae related to their posterior wall.
Source: Adapted from Dhingra's Textbook on Otorhinolaryngology.

is observed at a higher frequency in children suffering from allergic diseases, cigarette smoke exposure, and allergic rhinitis. Adenoid enlargement is diagnosed from a radiograph of the nasopharynx. Flexible nasal endoscopy aids in grading the extent of adenoid enlargement. The size is usually graded on a scale of I to IV.

Oropharynx

The tubulomuscular structure extending from the plane of the hard palate on the above to the plane of the hyoid bone below is termed as oropharynx. The oropharyngeal isthmus forms a communication between the oral cavity and the oropharynx. The palatine tonsil is anatomically located on the lateral wall of oropharynx in the tonsillar fossa. It is formed by the divergence of the anterior pillar or palatoglossal arch and the posterior pillar or palatopharyngeal arch.

Palatine Tonsil

Tonsil consists of a fibrous capsule that surrounds the entire structure and crypts made up of stratified squamous epithelium. These crypts increase the surface area for interaction with pathogens and facilitate immune responses. The bulk of the tonsil is composed of lymphoid tissue, which contains numerous immune cells including lymphocytes and macrophages. Tonsils have extensive blood supply predominantly from the external carotid artery tributaries. The glossopharyngeal and vagus nerves form the major nerve supply.

Physiological role of tonsils: Tonsils play a role in local immunity and surveillance. The tonsillar epithelium comprises specialized antigen-presenting M cells and micropores. Antigenic materials are presented to lymphoid follicles located in the subepithelial layer. The germinal center of the follicle is rich in B lymphocytes and the mantle zone is rich in large lymphocytes. B cells transform into plasma cells on exposure to stimulus and produce antibodies. The tonsillar macrophages carry out the function of phagocytosis.

Laryngopharynx/Hypopharynx

The terminal part of the pharynx, developing as a continuation of the oropharynx, is known as laryngopharynx. The structure is limited superiorly by the plane passing from the body of the hyoid bone to the posterior pharyngeal wall and the inferior limit is formed by the lower border of the cricoid cartilage. The hypopharynx continues as the esophagus at the level of cricoid cartilage.

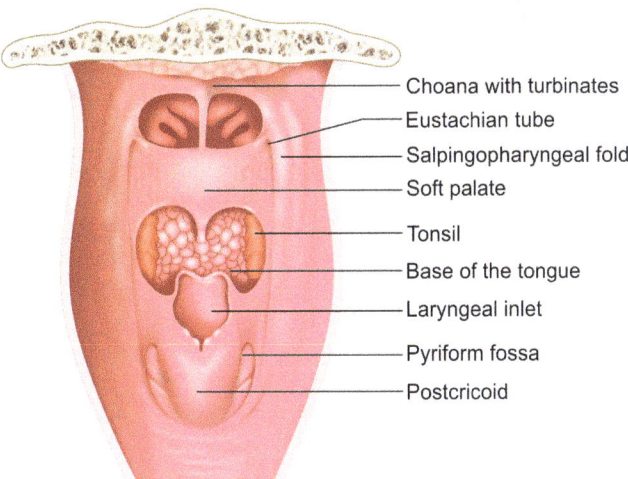

Fig. 8: Anatomical relations of nasopharynx, oropharynx, and laryngopharynx—pharynx reflected from behind.

Clinically, the hypopharynx is subdivided into three regions (**Fig. 8**):
1. Pyriform sinus
2. Postcricoid region
3. Posterior pharyngeal wall

Laryngopharyngeal Physiology

The laryngopharynx is composed of cartilages. The cricoid cartilage, along with the posterior cricoarytenoid muscles, work in synchrony to increase the glottic aperture. This coordinated function increases the cross-sectional area for airflow and plays an important role in preventing collapse of the laryngeal inlet during quiet spontaneous breathing.

■ CRITICAL OPENING PRESSURE OF UPPER AIRWAYS

The critical opening pressure is necessary to maintain the patency of the eustachian tube. This is the pressure threshold required to open the eustachian tube during air descent or mountain climbing, allowing air to flow into the middle ear (**Fig. 9**). When the pressure difference is too high, the tube may not open easily, leading to discomfort.

Critical Opening Pressure in the Larynx

The cricothyroid muscle is activated by positive pressure in the airway, regardless of the respiratory rate. The speed at which the airway pressure changes is important in triggering the cricothyroid muscle, with a critical level measured at around 30 cm H_2O per second. This opening pressure

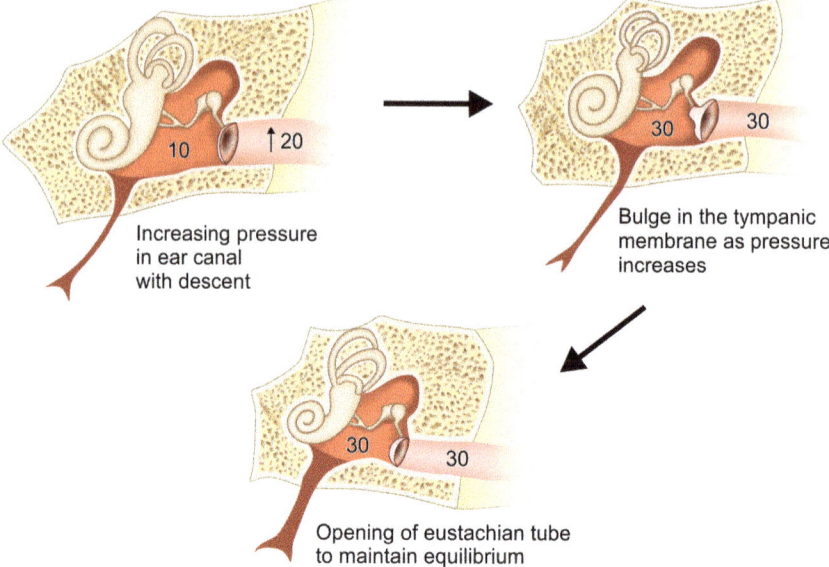

Fig. 9: Pressure changes in the middle ear cavity and critical opening pressure in the eustachian tube.

helps decrease airway resistance and shorten the duration of exhalation. The activation threshold of the cricothyroid muscle decreases in conditions of high carbon dioxide levels (hypercapnia) and increases in states of low carbon dioxide levels (hypocapnia).

Normal Defense Mechanisms of Upper Airways

The nose has efficient defense mechanisms that filter, humidify, and adjust the temperature. An adult on an average breathes 500 cubic feet of air each day. The nose filters the air we breathe from dust, bacteria, and viruses before it reaches the lungs **(Table 2)**.

■ SUMMARY

The nose exhibits a complex anatomy, comprising an osteocartilaginous framework, muscles, and skin, with external and internal components including nasal bones, cartilages, and the nasal septum. Turbinates and meatus further divide the nasal cavity, allowing for functions, such as respiration, air conditioning, filtration, and olfaction.

Air-filled cavities called paranasal sinuses surround the nasal cavity and play a vital role in air conditioning, voice resonance, and protection. The ostiomeatal unit regulates sinus drainage. The study of structure of the ear is clinically divided into external, middle, and inner parts.

TABLE 2: Summary of defensive mechanisms of upper airways.	
Upper airways	**Defensive mechanism**
Nasal vibrissae	Trap large particulate matter
Mucosal blanket	Trap finer particles, bacteria, pollen up to 6.6 µm
Eddy currents and air stream in nasal cycle	The adenoids respond immunologically when the air currents are impacted upon them
Mucosal blanket	Prevents dryness and damage of cilia
Sneeze reflex	Helps clear the nasal passages of foreign matter
Muramidase/lysozyme, IgA, IgE, and interferon in nasal secretions	Kills bacteria and viruses, immunity against respiratory infection
Adenoids and tonsils	Form the first-line defense gateway against pathogens that are ingested or inhaled
Eustachian tube	Maintains pressure equilibrium in the middle ear cavity
(IgA: immunoglobulin A; IgE: immunoglobulin E)	

The external structure is formed by the auricle and the auditory canal, while the middle ear cavity contains ossicles. The eustachian tube opens into the middle ear. Cochlea comprises the major portion of the inner ear. The physiological role of hearing and balance is chiefly carried out by the cochlea and the semicircular canals. The pressure changes in the middle ear can be balanced by techniques like the maneuver of Valsalva.

The pharynx is read under three divisions, namely (1) nasopharynx, (2) oropharynx, and (3) laryngopharynx. It plays a vital role in immune defense and airway maintenance, with each region having specific functions. For example, the nasopharynx houses adenoids for immune function, while the oropharynx contains palatine tonsils for local immunity.

■ KEY POINTS

- *Role of Upper Airways in Allergic Rhinitis:* The upper airways are crucial in the manifestation of allergic rhinitis, a prevalent chronic condition affecting both children and adults. Understanding the anatomy and physiology of the upper airways is essential for effective prevention and treatment strategies.
- *Anatomy and Function of the Nose:* The nose, composed of both external and internal structures, plays multiple roles including respiration, air-conditioning, protection of the lower airways, vocal resonance, and olfaction. Its intricate structure, including the nasal septum, turbinates, and meatuses, is vital for these functions.

- *Physiology of the Paranasal Sinuses:* The paranasal sinuses, including the maxillary, ethmoid, frontal, and sphenoid sinuses, serve functions such as air-conditioning, voice resonance, and protection of delicate structures in the orbit and cranium. Ventilation of these sinuses is synchronized with nasal respiration.
- *Ear Anatomy and Physiology:* The ear, divided into external, middle, and inner parts, is responsible for hearing and balance. The tympanic membrane, ossicles, and cochlea are key components involved in sound transmission and balance maintenance, with the vestibular system playing a critical role in spatial orientation and equilibrium.
- *Critical Opening Pressure in the Eustachian Tube and Larynx:* The concept of critical opening pressure is important for maintaining the patency of the Eustachian tube and the larynx. Proper functioning of these structures is crucial for equalizing pressure in the middle ear and preventing collapse of the larynx during respiration.

SUGGESTED READING

1. Ball M, Hossain M, Padalia D. Anatomy, Airway. 2023 Jul 25. In: StatPearls [Internet]. Treasure Island (FL): StatPearls Publishing; 2024.
2. Barrett KE, Barman SM, Brooks HL, Yuan JJ. Ganong's Review of Medical Physiology, 26th edition. New York: McGraw-Hill Education; 2019.
3. Dhingra PL, Dhingra S, Dhingra D. Diseases of Ear, Nose and Throat & Head and Neck Surgery, 6th edition. Gurugram: Elsevier; 2014.
4. Drake RL, Vogl W, Mitchell AW, Gray H. Gray's Anatomy for Students, 2nd edition. Philadelphia: Churchill Livingstone/Elsevier; 2010.
5. Hall JE, Hall ME. Guyton and Hall Textbook of Medical Physiology, 14th edition. Philadelphia, PA: Elsevier; 2020.
6. Horiuchi M, Sasaki CT. Cricothyroid muscle in respiration. Ann Otol Rhinol Laryngol. 1978;87(3 Pt 1):386-91.
7. Mnatsakanian A, Heil JR, Sharma S. Anatomy, Head and Neck: Adenoids. In: StatPearls [Internet]. Treasure Island (FL): StatPearls Publishing; 2024.
8. Nathan RA. Nathan RA. The burden of allergic rhinitis. Allergy Asthma Proc. 2007;28(1):3-9.
9. Sahin-Yilmaz A, Naclerio RM. Anatomy and physiology of the upper airway. Proc Am Thorac Soc. 2011;8(1):31-9.
10. Sasaki CT, Weaver EM. Physiology of the larynx. Am J Med. 1997;103(5A):9S-18S.
11. Snow Jr JB, Ballenger JJ. Ballenger's Otorhinolaryngology Head and Neck Surgery, 16th edition. Hamilton, Ontario: BC Decker Inc; 2003.
12. Wani TM, Bissonnette B, Engelhardt T, Buchh B, Arnous H, AlGhamdi F, et al. The pediatric airway: historical concepts, new findings, and what matters. Int J Pediatr Otorhinolaryngol. 2019;121:29-33.

CHAPTER 2

Rhinitis Classification

Hima Mathews P

■ INTRODUCTION

Rhinitis refers to the inflammation of the nasal mucosa, which results in a combination of symptoms which include nasal itching, sneezing, anterior or posterior rhinorrhea, and nasal obstruction. Sinusitis is characterized by inflammation of the paranasal sinuses. Rhinosinusitis occurs as these structures are in close proximity and contiguity, resulting in their simultaneous involvement. Most common cause of rhinitis is allergic rhinitis and pathophysiology of nonallergic rhinitis (NAR) is still remain unclear. Chronic rhinitis has a significant impact on productivity and quality of life.

■ CAUSES OF RHINITIS

The causes of rhinitis are given in **Box 1**.

■ DEFINITION OF CHRONIC RHINITS

Chronic rhinitis is characterized by inflammation of nasal mucosa, which causes symptoms such as nasal blockage, rhinorrhea (anterior or posterior), sneezing, and itching in the nose or eyes. Any two of the above-mentioned nasal symptoms has to be present for a minimum of 1 hour per day for at least 12 weeks per year **(Flowchart 1)**.

Chronic rhinitis is divided into four major categories:
1. Allergic rhinitis
2. Infectious rhinitis
3. Noninfectious rhinitis
4. Mixed rhinitis

Allergic Rhinitis

Allergic rhinitis, which was thought to be a localized disease initially, is now considered to be a part of a generalized respiratory system disease as per the newer research data. The upper and lower respiratory tract have several physiological, functional, and immunological similarities.

Allergic rhinitis occurs after exposure to an allergen in a prior sensitized individual, and is mediated by immunoglobulin E (IgE)-mediated type 1 hypersensitivity. Even though allergic rhinitis does not have a significant impact on morbidity and mortality rates, due to high prevalence of around

> **BOX 1:** Causes of rhinitis.
>
> *Allergic rhinitis:*
> - Seasonal
> - Perennial
> - Perennial with seasonal exacerbation
> - Local allergic rhinitis
>
> *Nonallergic rhinitis:*
> - Infectious
> - Idiopathic
> - Nonallergic rhinitis with eosinophilia
> - Drug-induced
> - Hormonal
> - Atrophic
> - Gustatory
> - Toxic/occupational
> - Autoimmune:
>   – Granulomatosis with polyangiitis
>   – Eosinophilic granulomatosis with polyangiitis
>   – Sarcoid
>
> *Anatomic:*
> - Adenoid hypertrophy
> - Foreign body
> - Choanal atresia
> - Tumors
> - Cerebrospinal fluid leaks
>
> *Rhinosinusitis:*
> - Chronic with and without nasal polyps
> - Cystic fibrosis
> - Primary ciliary dyskinesia
> - Fungal/allergic fungal rhinosinusitis
>
> *Source:* Hellings PW, Klimek L, Cingi C, Agache I, Akdis C, Bachert C, et al. Non-allergic rhinitis: Position paper of the European Academy of Allergy and Clinical Immunology. Allergy. 2017;72(11):1657-65.

400 million people globally, its burden on individuals and society is substantial compared to many other diseases.

Allergic rhinitis can be classified into:
- Seasonal
- Perennial
- Perennial with seasonal exacerbation
- Local allergic rhinitis (LAR)

The new terminology "intermittent and persistent allergic rhinitis" was introduced in the 2001 Allergic Rhinitis and its Impact on Asthma (ARIA) guidelines.

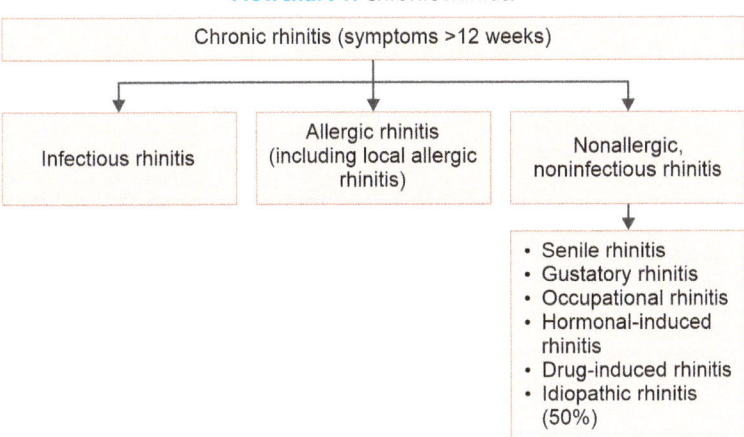

Flowchart 1: Chronic rhinitis.

Source: Wise SK, Lin SY, Toskala E, Orlandi RR, Akdis CA, Alt JA, et al. International Consensus Statement on Allergy and Rhinology: Allergic Rhinitis. Int Forum Allergy Rhinol. 2018;8(2):108-352.

Seasonal Versus Perennial Allergic Rhinitis

"Seasonal allergic rhinitis" is caused by outdoor allergens, mostly pollens. "Perennial allergic rhinitis" occurs on exposure to indoor allergens and persists throughout the year. Examples of indoor allergens include dust mites, cockroach, molds, and animal dander. As there could be varying degree of exposure to indoor allergens with intermittent exacerbations, the classification of seasonal and perennial allergic rhinitis could not explain all clinical scenarios. For example, house dust mite an indoor allergen can cause intermittent allergic rhinitis also. To overcome this, *ARIA* introduced a new classification system considering the duration, intensity, and frequency of the symptoms.

Symptoms occurring for <4 days/week or lasting for <4 consecutive weeks is classified as intermittent rhinitis and symptoms persisting for >4 days/week, for a minimum of 4 consecutive weeks as persistent rhinitis.

Allergic rhinitis is classified as "mild" when symptoms are not bothersome and do not impact everyday activities or sleep and moderate to severe if it affects daily routine **(Flowchart 2)**.

Local Allergic Rhinitis

Local allergic rhinitis, also called entropy, is a specific type of allergic rhinitis. It is characterized by a localized type 2 inflammation of the nasal mucosa and it includes the production of specific IgE antibodies, but without any evidence of generalized atopy. This means that allergen prick testing for common aeroallergens yields negative results, and serum-specific IgE (sIgE) antibodies

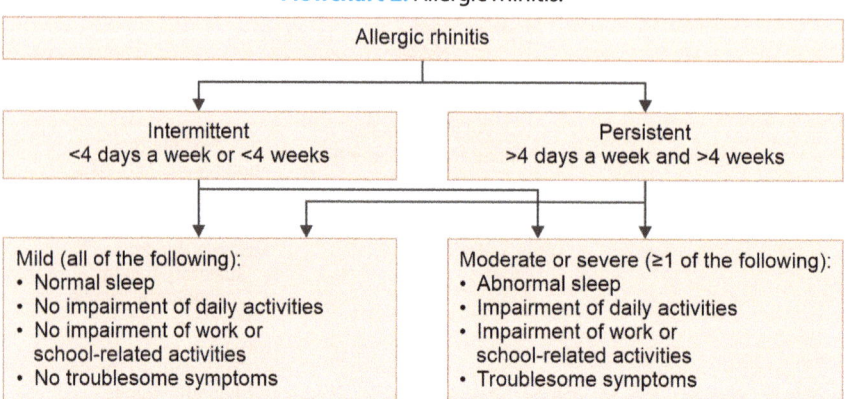

Flowchart 2: Allergic rhinitis.

Source: Eiwegger T, Soyka MB. Allergic rhinitis. In: Leung DYM, Akdis CA, Bacharier LB, Cunningham-Rundles C, Sicherer SH, Sampson HA (Eds). Pediatric Allergy: Principles and Practice, 4th edition. New York: Elsevier; 2020. pp. 135-47.

cannot be detected. Prevalence is still unclear as this is often underdiagnosed and it denotes a specific category previously referred to as "nonallergic rhinitis with eosinophilia syndrome" (NARES). The pathophysiology is distinguished by the localized production of sIgE and is also characterized by Th2 inflammatory infiltration. History of allergic rhinitis like symptoms, when exposed to natural airborne allergens are present and the diagnosis of LAR can be confirmed by detecting sIgE in the nasal mucosa or positive nasal allergen challenge test or both.

Infectious Rhinitis

Infectious rhinitis could be acute and chronic types which can be caused by both viruses and bacteria. The presence of physical findings and the duration of symptoms are crucial factors in distinguishing various types of rhinitis. Indicators of a noninfectious cause include nasal irritation and sneezing, but signs of mucosal inflammation and rhinorrhea can be present in both infectious and noninfectious rhinitis.

Nonallergic Rhinitis

Nonallergic rhinitis accounts for approximately 25% of all cases of rhinitis. Pathophysiology of this condition is still not well understood, and there are no specific diagnostic tests available. It is a group of heterogeneous syndromes that share similar clinical features including nasal congestion and rhinorrhea, without itching of nose, pharynx or eyes, sneezing, nasal polyps, eczema, or lower respiratory tract symptoms. Approximately 50% of people with NAR have symptoms for which the underlying cause is unknown, and are referred to as idiopathic rhinitis. Clinical subgroups can be characterized by features such as the absence of allergy or specific triggers. The existing research indicates that nociceptor and autonomic nerve dysfunction are key factors in all types of NAR.

Nonallergic Rhinopathy (Idiopathic Nonallergic Rhinitis)

This entity was formerly known as "vasomotor rhinitis" and it is defined by nasal symptoms that are induced by environmental factors, such as potent odors, variations in temperature, humidity, or barometric pressure. These symptoms usually occur without nasal and palatal itching or significant sneezing. Nonallergic rhinopathy is a diagnosis that is made by ruling out other possible causes of rhinitis. Formerly known as "vasomotor rhinitis," this condition was renamed due to insufficient data supporting a vascular etiology.

Senile Rhinitis

Senile or geriatric rhinitis primarily affects older people and onset of symptoms is late compared to other forms of rhinitis. The symptoms manifest as watery rhinorrhea that becomes more severe when the patient is exposed to specific triggers, such as certain foods, smells, or irritants in the surroundings. The aging process in the nasal cavity leads to neurological, hormonal, mucosal, olfactory, and histologic changes that affect the structure and function of the nose. The symptoms are believed to be caused by neurogenic dysregulation. Effectiveness of ipratropium bromide, an anticholinergic drug, reduces the intensity and duration of rhinorrhea in these patients which support the pathophysiology.

Drug-induced Rhinitis

Drug-induced rhinitis can arise as a result of using various medications, such as nonsteroidal anti-inflammatory drugs, antihypertensives, phosphodiesterase-5 inhibitors, and cocaine. Drug-induced rhinitis is commonly classified into three distinct categories: (1) neurogenic, (2) inflammatory, and (3) idiopathic. While many drugs include rhinitis as a potential side effect, the most significant ones are antihypertensive medications which induce rhinitis through neurogenic mechanisms by suppressing the release of norepinephrine, resulting in congestion and rhinorrhea due to the dominance of the parasympathetic system in the nasal mucosa. Rhinitis medicamentosa occurs due to excess use of topical decongestants for >3–5 days, causing a rebound nonallergic vascular congestion.

Gustatory Rhinitis

Gustatory rhinitis is the nasal response to the consumption of certain foods, such as spicy meals and alcohol. Its primary distinguishing feature is its trigger, and it frequently overlaps with senile rhinitis. It is thought to be caused by a gustatory reflex linked to hyperactive nerve endings in the aerodigestive tract.

Hormonal Rhinitis

Hormonal rhinitis is characterized by the occurrence of nasal congestion and rhinorrhea caused by female hormones. Pregnancy is the most prevalent cause and symptoms abate toward the conclusion of pregnancy. Hormone-induced rhinitis is characterized by nasal congestion caused by increased levels of estrogen and progesterone. Estrogens cause increased blood flow in the nasal blood vessels, resulting in nasal congestion and excessive nasal mucus production. Beta-estradiol and progesterone enhance the manifestation of histamine H1-receptors on human nasal epithelium and microvascular endothelial cells, leading to the stimulation of eosinophil migration and/or degranulation.

Occupational Rhinitis

Occupational rhinitis refers to nasal inflammation that causes symptoms, such as nasal congestion, sneezing, runny nose, itching, and excessive mucus production, caused by factors in the workplace environment, rather than external stimuli encountered outside of work. Occupational rhinitis is classified as a type of "work-related rhinitis," which also includes work-exacerbated rhinitis. Work-exacerbated rhinitis refers to preexisting or concurrent rhinitis that is aggravated by occupational exposures. Work-related rhinitis could be either caused by work (occupational rhinitis) or exacerbated by work (work-exacerbated rhinitis).

■ ACUTE SINUSITIS

"Acute sinusitis is an inflammation of the paranasal sinuses and the nasal cavity lasting no longer than 4 weeks characterized by purulent nasal discharge (anterior, posterior, or both) accompanied by nasal obstruction, facial pain-pressure-fullness, or both."

The term acute sinusitis and acute rhinosinusitis has been used interchangeably.

■ RHINOSINUSITIS

Rhinosinusitis is a broad term for a number of different diseases, such as acute rhinosinusitis (ARS), chronic rhinosinusitis with nasal polyps (CRSwNP), and chronic rhinosinusitis without nasal polyps (CRSsNP).

Rhinosinusitis is defined as inflammation of the nose and the paranasal sinuses characterized by two or more symptom complex given here.

One of which should be either nasal blockage/obstruction/congestion or nasal discharge (anterior/posterior nasal drip).
- ± Facial pain/pressure
- ± Reduction or loss of smell (or cough in children)

And either endoscopic signs of nasal polyps, and/or mucopurulent discharge primarily from middle meatus and/or edema/mucosal obstruction primarily in middle meatus

And/or CT changes: Mucosal changes within the ostiomeatal complex and/or sinuses.

Clinical Definition of Rhinosinusitis

Clinical definition of rhinosinusitis is given in **Flowchart 3**.

Viral Rhinosinusitis

Viral rhinosinusitis is defined as presence of signs and symptoms of rhinosinusitis ≤10 days without worsening.

Acute Bacterial Rhinosinusitis

Presumption of bacterial rhinosinusitis to be made when signs or symptoms of ARS either does not improve within ≥10 days or worsen within 10 days after an initial improvement (double worsening).

Flowchart 3: Acute rhinosinusitis.

```
                    Acute rhinosinusitis (ARS)
                    ┌────────────┴────────────┐
                  Adults                   Children
                    │                         │
            Definition: Sudden onset of two or
                    more symptoms:
```

Adults	Children
One of which should be either: • Nasal blockage/obstruction/congestion or • Nasal discharge (anterior/posterior nasal drip) • ± Facial pain/pressure • ± Reduction or loss of smell	• Nasal blockage/obstruction/congestion • Or discolored nasal discharge • Or cough (daytime and night-time)

For <12 weeks

Source: Grayson JW, Hopkins C, Mori E, Senior B, Harvey RJ. Contemporary Classification of Chronic Rhinosinusitis Beyond Polyps vs No Polyps: A Review. JAMA Otolaryngol Head Neck Surg. 2020;146(9):831-8.

TABLE 1: Features of CRSwNP and CRSsNP.	
CRSwNP	• Th2 inflammation with eosinophilic predominance • Nasal block and anosmia with good response to steroids • Associated with asthma
CRSsNP	• Th1 inflammation with neutrophilic predominance • Facial pain and postnasal drip with good response to macrolides • Less associated with asthma

(CRSsNP: chronic rhinosinusitis without nasal polyps; CRSwNP: chronic rhinosinusitis with nasal polyps)
Source: Grayson JW, Hopkins C, Mori E, Senior B, Harvey RJ. Contemporary Classification of Chronic Rhinosinusitis Beyond Polyps vs No Polyps: A Review. JAMA Otolaryngol Head Neck Surg. 2020;146(9):831-8.

Recurrent Acute Rhinosinusitis

Recurrent acute rhinosinusitis (RARS) is defined as ≥4 episodes per year with symptom-free intervals.

Chronic Rhinosinusitis

Chronic rhinosinusitis (CRS) is defined as the presence of symptoms of ARS that remains for 12 weeks or more.

Based on the current guideline, CRS is characterized phenotypically depending on the presence of nasal polyps: CRSwNP and CRSsNP **(Table 1)**.

Present recommendations categorize CRS into primary and secondary forms. Primary CRS is currently defined as a primary inflammatory condition that specifically affects the airway or respiratory system, without involving any other parts of the body **(Flowchart 4)**.

Secondary CRS indicates the presence of either local or systemic disease that is responsible for the alterations in the sinuses. Diffuse disease refers to a condition that is not limited to a specific anatomical area. The mechanism for diffuse disease suggests that there is another process occurring alongside CRS, and this process may involve inflammatory (often autoimmune), mechanical (mucociliary), or immunodeficiency **(Flowchart 5)**.

■ ALLERGIC CONJUNCTIVITIS

Allergic conjunctivitis is an inflammation of conjunctiva due to an allergic or hypersensitivity reaction. Over 95% of individuals with seasonal or perennial allergic conjunctivitis also have allergic rhinitis, and the term "allergic rhinoconjunctivitis" is sometimes used interchangeably with allergic conjunctivitis.

Flowchart 4: Primary CRS.

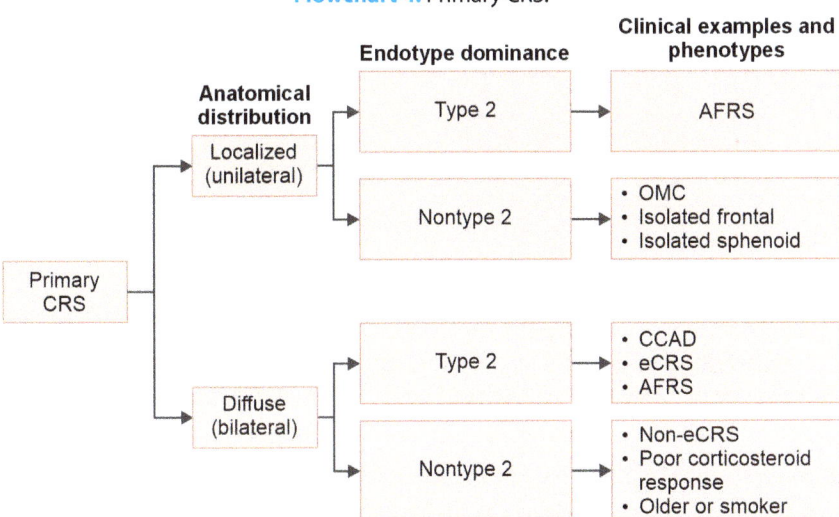

(AFRS: allergic fungal rhinosinusitis; CCAD: central compartment atopic disease; CRS: chronic rhinosinusitis; eCRS: eosinophilic CRS; OMC: ostiomeatal complex)
Source: Fokkens WJ, Lund VJ, Hopkins C, Hellings PW, Kern R, Reitsma S, et al. European Position Paper on Rhinosinusitis and Nasal Polyps 2020. Rhinology. 2020;58(Suppl S29):1-464.

Flowchart 5: Secondary chronic rhinosinusitis (CRS).

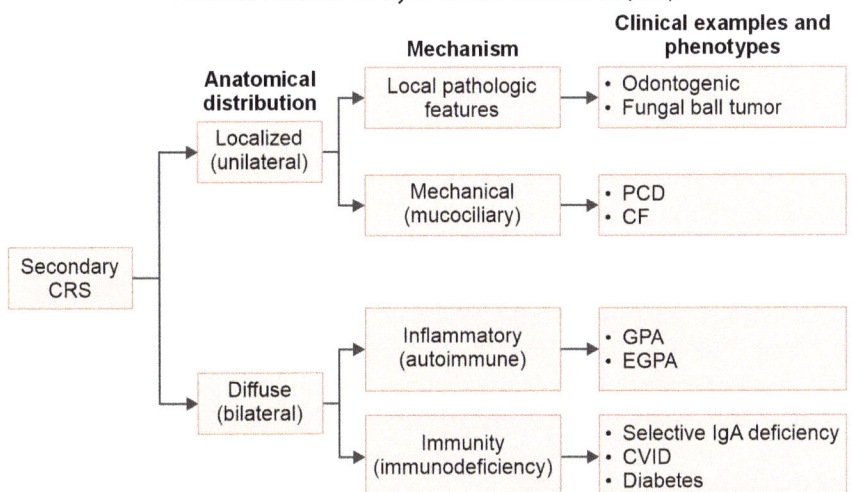

(CF: cystic fibrosis; CVID: common variable immunodeficiency; EGPA: eosinophilic granulomatosis with polyangiitis; GPA: granulomatosis with polyangiitis; IgA: Immunoglobulin A; PCD: primary ciliary dyskinesia)
Source: Fokkens WJ, Lund VJ, Hopkins C, Hellings PW, Kern R, Reitsma S, et al. European Position Paper on Rhinosinusitis and Nasal Polyps 2020. Rhinology. 2020;58(Suppl S29):1-464.

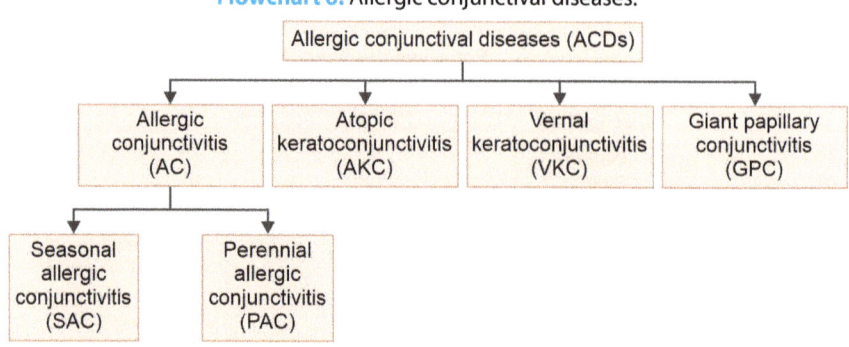

Flowchart 6: Allergic conjunctival diseases.

Source: Riggioni Víquez S, Riggioni Víquez C, Ribó González P. Diagnosis and Management of Allergic Conjunctivitis. Curr Treat Options Allergy. 2018;5(5):256-65.

Classification of Allergic Conjunctivitis

Allergic rhinoconjuctivitis is linked to other respiratory allergies, i.e., sinusitis, asthma, and otitis media, and share a common etiology. Allergic conjunctivitis is caused by a complex allergen-triggered inflammation of the conjunctiva. Seasonal allergic conjunctivitis includes allergic conjunctival diseases without proliferative changes, where symptoms appear in a seasonal manner and in perennial allergic conjunctivitis symptoms persist throughout the year **(Flowchart 6)**.

Vernal Keratoconjunctivitis

Vernal keratoconjunctivitis (VKC) is an allergic inflammation of the conjunctiva with seasonal exacerbation resulting from a complex pathophysiology involving IgE and cell-mediated immune mechanisms.

Based on clinical presentation, it can be classified into three forms:
1. *Palpebral VKC:* Primarily affects the upper tarsal conjunctiva and is characterized by significant corneal involvement from the close apposition between the inflamed conjunctiva and the corneal epithelium.
2. *Limbal VKC:* It affects the bulbar conjunctiva| in the palpebral area.
3. *Mixed VKC:* It is a subtype that exhibits a combination of features seen in both palpebral and limbal disease.

Atopic Keratoconjunctivitis

It is a chronic inflammatory disease of the eye with a multifactorial origin and the etiology still remains unclear. However, various factors including atopic dermatitis (present in >90% of cases), exposure to allergen, and genetic predisposition play an important role. It is a potentially serious condition causing significant visual morbidity.

Giant Papillary Conjunctivitis

It is characterized by the formation of giant papillae which usually occur due to mechanical irritation of the palpebral conjunctiva due to ocular foreign bodies such as contact lenses, ocular prostheses, cyanoacrylate glue, and sutures. The occurrence of giant papillary conjunctivitis can be ascribed to ocular foreign bodies, which could harbor allergens or cause damage to the ocular tissue, allowing allergens to enter.

Otitis Media

Otitis media includes acute otitis media (AOM), chronic suppurative otitis media (CSOM), and otitis media with effusion (OME).

Acute otitis media: It is an acute infection of the middle ear, causing inflammation and accumulation of purulent fluid in the middle ear. It is characterized by acute onset of symptoms (fever, ear pain, or ear discharge), associated with middle ear effusion diagnosed by bulging tympanic membrane/decreased mobility/air fluid level behind the membrane, associated with features of middle ear inflammation indicated by erythema of tympanic membrane.

Nonsevere AOM: AOM with mild otalgia and a temperature <39°C

Severe AOM: AOM with moderate-to-severe otalgia or a fever >39°C

Recurrent AOM: >3 well-documented separate AOM episodes in the past 6 months, or 2–4 episodes in the past 12 months with at least on episode in the past 6 months.

Uncomplicated AOM: AOM without otorrhea.

Persistent AOM: Persistent signs/symptoms of AOM during antimicrobial therapy and/or relapse of AOM 1 month after completing an antibiotic regimen.

Otitis media with effusion: Chronic accumulation of nonpurulent effusion or mucus within the middle ear cleft is known as OME. There are no signs or symptoms of an acute ear infection associated with the fluid collection. The diagnosis can be made based on one or more of the following findings: decreased movement of the tympanic membrane when examined with a pneumatic otoscope, decreased movement of the tympanic membrane when tested with tympanometry, an opaque tympanic membrane, or the presence of a visible air-fluid interface behind the tympanic membrane when examined with an otoscope. OME that lasts for at least 3 months has significantly lower rates of natural resolution compared to new-onset OME or OME following an episode of AOM.

Chronic suppurative otitis media: Chronic suppurative otitis media is characterized by chronic infection of the mucosa of the middle ear cleft, characterized by continuous or intermittent discharge through a tympanic membrane perforation. There is no consensus on the specific length of time that ear discharge should persist in order to make a diagnosis but usually considered as lasting for at least months. CSOM refers to the ongoing inflammation of the middle ear or mastoid cavity. Alternate terms for this condition are "chronic otitis media", chronic mastoiditis, and chronic tympanomastoiditis. CSOM typically arises as a consequence of prolonged AOM with perforation.

Chronic suppurative otitis media is classified into two main types:
1. *Atticoantral type*, which is also known as "attic or marginal perforation," affects the pars flaccida or posterosuperior marginal quadrant. This is referred to as an "unsafe" type of CSOM as it can lead to dangerous intracranial complications, most often caused by cholesteatoma. There will be a scanty foul smelling discharge and moderate-to-serious hearing loss, which could lead to permanent deafness.
2. *Tubotympanic type*, also known as central tympanic perforation, involves the pars tensa. It is the "safe" type because it is less likely to cause serious complications like meningitis and brain abscesses. Intermittent episodes of profuse mucopurulent discharge occur and it can cause gradually progressive conductive hearing loss. It is often triggered by respiratory tract infection.

■ SUMMARY

Allergic rhinitis is one of the most common inflammatory airway diseases with high worldwide prevalence. Distinction between allergic and nonallergic forms of rhinitis is essential for treatment and preventing complications, but most of the cases it is not easy to differentiate between these two entities. Rhinosinusitis and rhinitis is always used interchangeably nowadays as they coexist in most of the scenarios. Allergic rhinitis is almost always accompanied by allergic conjunctivitis and represents different manifestation of the same inflammatory process. Otitis media can occur in association with rhinitis, and diagnosis of the primary cause leading to otitis media should be addressed to avoid complication.

■ KEY POINTS

- Allergic rhinitis is an IgE-mediated, type 1 hypersensitivity, resulting from exposure to an allergen in a sensitized individual.
- Allergic rhinitis is a systemic inflammatory disease, even though initially it was considered as a localized disease.

- Knowledge about the classification of rhinitis is essential to decide on further treatment and to prevent complications.
- Allergic rhinitis is almost always associated with allergic conjunctivitis.
- Rhinosinusitis and otitis media represent the spectrum of coexisting morbidities as well as the complications of rhinitis which could be prevented with if rhinitis is addressed early with appropriate treatment and follow-up.

SUGGESTED READING

1. Baab S, Le PH, Gurnani B, Kinzer EE. Allergic Conjunctivitis. In: StatPearls [Internet]. Treasure Island (FL): StatPearls Publishing; 2024.
2. DeBoer DL, Kwon E. Acute Sinusitis. In: StatPearls [Internet]. Treasure Island (FL): StatPearls Publishing; 2024.
3. Eiwegger T, Soyka MB. Allergic rhinitis. In: Leung DYM, Akdis CA, Bacharier LB, Cunningham-Rundles C, Sicherer SH, Sampson HA (Eds). Pediatric Allergy: Principles and Practice, 4th edition. New York: Elsevier; 2020. pp. 135-47.
4. Fokkens WJ, Lund VJ, Hopkins C, Hellings PW, Kern R, Reitsma S, et al. European Position Paper on Rhinosinusitis and Nasal Polyps 2020. Rhinology. 2020;58(Suppl S29):1-464.
5. Goniotakis I, Perikleous E, Fouzas S, Steiropoulos P, Paraskakis E. A Clinical Approach of Allergic Rhinitis in Children. Children (Basel). 2023;10(9):1571.
6. Grayson JW, Hopkins C, Mori E, Senior B, Harvey RJ. Contemporary Classification of Chronic Rhinosinusitis Beyond Polyps vs No Polyps: A Review. JAMA Otolaryngol Head Neck Surg. 2020;146(9):831-8.
7. Gupta N, Moitra S, Nagarajan S. Comprehensive Textbook of Allergy: Striking the Right Balance, 1st edition. New Delhi: Jaypee Brothers Medical Publishers; 2024.
8. Hellings PW, Klimek L, Cingi C, Agache I, Akdis C, Bachert C, et al. Non-allergic rhinitis: Position paper of the European Academy of Allergy and Clinical Immunology. Allergy. 2017;72(11):1657-65.
9. Lieberthal AS, Carroll AE, Chonmaitree T, Ganiats TG, Hoberman A, Jackson MA, et al. The diagnosis and management of acute otitis media. Pediatrics. 2013;131(3):e964-99. Erratum in: Pediatrics. 2014;133(2):346.
10. Morris P. Chronic suppurative otitis media. BMJ Clin Evid. 2012;2012:0507.
11. Riggioni Víquez S, Riggioni Víquez C, Ribó González P. Diagnosis and Management of Allergic Conjunctivitis. Curr Treat Options Allergy. 2018;5(5):256-65.
12. Scadding GK, Smith PK, Blaiss M, Roberts G, Hellings PW, Gevaert P, et al. Allergic Rhinitis in Childhood and the New EUFOREA Algorithm. Front Allergy. 2021;2:706589.
13. Schilder AG, Chonmaitree T, Cripps AW, Rosenfeld RM, Casselbrant ML, Haggard MP, et al. Otitis media. Nat Rev Dis Primers. 2016;2(1):16063.
14. Takamura E, Uchio E, Ebihara N, Ohno S, Ohashi Y, Okamoto S, et al. Japanese guidelines for allergic conjunctival diseases 2017. Allergol Int. 2017;66(2):220-9.
15. Vedantan PK, Nelson HS, Agashe SN, Mahesh PA, Katial R. Textbook of Allergy for the Clinician, 2nd edition. Boca Raton: CRC Press; 2021.
16. Wise SK, Lin SY, Toskala E, Orlandi RR, Akdis CA, Alt JA, et al International Consensus Statement on Allergy and Rhinology: Allergic Rhinitis. Int Forum Allergy Rhinol. 2018;8(2):108-352.

CHAPTER 3

Allergic Rhinitis: Pathophysiology

Soundarya M

■ INTRODUCTION

Allergic rhinitis (AR) has a complex pathophysiology with numerous etiological factors. It is an interplay between the allergenic triggers, genetic and epigenetic factors, irritants, and an abnormal immune mechanism in the upper respiratory tract. In the atopic march, AR appears in the latter end of the spectrum as compared to atopic dermatitis and food allergies which come earlier on.

■ ETIOLOGY

The etiology of AR includes the various causes which encompass both allergenic triggers as well as irritants in the genetically predisposed individual.

Genetics and Epigenetics

The expression of allergic diseases of the upper airways reflects an autosomal dominant pattern of inheritance with incomplete penetrance and is manifested as a tendency to respond to inhalant allergen exposure by producing high levels of allergen-specific immunoglobulin E (IgE). This response is moderated by immune response genes located within the major histocompatibility complex on chromosome 6. For this, there has been a lot of evidence over the last two decades furthering the understanding about the genetic linking of AR. This has surfaced in twin studies showing the heritable nature of the disease. The concordance rate for atopic dermatitis in identical twins is approximately 80%, which is much higher than the 20% concordance rate observed in fraternal twins. Heritability estimates calculations for AR show approximately 33–91% heritability risk.

The various gene loci that have been identified are mentioned in **Table 1**. The main functions of these loci are in immune regulation, function, and regulation of T cells, B cells, natural killer (NK) cells, immune mechanisms in airway epithelium, and in innate immunity pathways.

Epigenetics has also played a role in the pathogenesis of AR. Here studies have shown that the histone deacetylase is increased in patients with AR and inhibition of the same helps in improving symptoms of AR. The gene for histone deacetylase is *HDAC1* which is upregulated by interleukin 4 (IL4)

TABLE 1: Genes (identified till date) attributed to predisposition for allergic rhinitis.	
Chromosomes	Genes
19p13	MRPL4
11q13	C11orf30/LRRC32
5q22.1	• TSLP • TMEM232, SLCA25A46
6p21.32	HLA region (BTNL2, HLA-DPB1, HLA-DQA1, HLA-DQB1, HLA-DRB1, HLA-DRB3, HLA-DRB4, HLA-DRB5, TAP1, and TAP2)
11q13.5	C11orf30, LRRC32
1q23.3	AL590714.1, FCER1G
4q24	MANBA, NFKB1
10q24.32	ACTR1A, TMEM180
12q24.31	SPPL3, ACADS

in the nasal epithelium and hence plays a role in the pathophysiology of AR. Similarly, deoxyribonucleic acid (DNA) methylation changes which are inherited in an epigenetic pattern also play a role in AR. Changes in DNA methylation causing hypomethylation cause increased IL33 and IgE. Sublingual immunotherapy has been associated with changes in DNA methylation sites in immune regulatory cells, all suggesting that the DNA methylation plays a role in AR pathophysiology and can also be responsible for paternally transmitted genetic variants of AR. Another aspect in epigenetics is the role of microRNAs (miRNAs) in the pathophysiology of AR. These are small signaling peptides which regulate gene expression. Studies have shown that decreased expression of miRNA (miR-126 and miR-21) in neonatal leukocytes has been associated with the development of AR and upregulation of certain miRNA (498, 187, and 874) and downregulation of other miRNA (224, 255, and 126) are seen in patients with AR.

Allergens

Allergens are mainly antigenic molecules that trigger the nasal mucosal immune response. The main allergens are:
- *Aeroallergens:* The aeroallergens are the main and most common cause of true AR. The antigens are of 2–20 μm in size and easily enter the nose reaching the posterior nasal cavity. These molecules are primarily proteinaceous molecules and hence trigger an immune response. The following are the most common allergen:
    - *House dust mite:* The most common antigen that has been implicated in causing AR is the fecal particles of the house dust mite (bed mite—*Dermatophagoides pteronyssinus*, floor mite—*Dermatophagoides*

farinae and *Blomia* spp.). The mites are not of the insect family and instead belong to the arachnid family. The main allergenic component of the house dust mites is its fecal particles which are of size 30 μm and are easily airborne. The important antigenic components of this allergen are the Der p 1, Der p 2, and Der p 23. The mite sheds nearly 1,000 fecal particles in its lifetime (approximately 3 months). These fecal pellets are heavier than most other allergens and tend to become airborne when disturbed for example during dusting and settle within half an hour. Apart from the fecal particles, parts of the chitinous exoskeleton also have allergenic properties. Once these particles are airborne, they are easily inhaled and enter the nasal/bronchial mucosa where they trigger the Th2 response.

- *Cockroach:* The household cockroach is one of the common pests and also contributes to significant allergenic sensitization worldwide. Of the many species, the American cockroach (*Periplaneta americana*) and the German cockroach (*Blattella germanica*) are most commonly associated with allergies. The main cockroach allergens are the gut proteins and proteases, lipocalins, tropomyosin, and troponins. The sources of these proteins are the cockroach frass, eggs, particles of the cuticle/chitin, and saliva. The size of these allergens is 7-10 μm and is easily airborne. Being heavy, these particles settle down and are again airborne when disturbed during cleaning and dusting. The main antigenic components are Bla g 1, Bla g 2, and Bla g 7. The amount of antigen in the household dust is measured as an indicator of the extent of exposure to cockroach antigen. A level of >2 U/g of dust has been known to cause sensitization and a risk factor for allergy and asthma.
- *Mold:* There are five major species of fungi which are implicated in the causation of allergy—Oomycetes, Zygomycetes, ascomycetes, basidiomycetes, and Deuteromycetes that are ubiquitous in nature. The spores of these various fungi are released in millions into the air and are significantly allergenic particles. These fungi grow in damp and warm conditions; hence, rotting wood, soggy leaves, damp walls, carpets, old furniture, undersurface of sinks and basins, bathrooms, storage areas of air coolers, and humidifiers are perfect locations. The spores are very small ~5-10 μm in diameter and are dispersed in large numbers. Being very light, they are dispersed far and wide as well as are very resistant to weather conditions, surviving unfavorable conditions for a long time. Among the fungi, spores of *Rhizopus, Mucor, Aspergillus, Candida,* and *Penicillium* are the most common fungi responsible for sensitization. In the upper airway, these spores once inhaled can lodge in the nasal cavities as well as in the paranasal

sinuses and trigger the allergic inflammatory response as well as produce invasive disease.
- *Pollens:* Pollens are the male gametes in plants, which are small structures that result in seed production after fertilization with the female gametocyte. Pollen grains are produced by both wind pollinated and insect pollinated plants; however, the wind pollinated plant pollens are much smaller and lighter unlike the insect pollinated plant pollens. Hence, the pollens of the wind pollinated plants are the main allergenic pollens. The size of these pollens is around 20–50 µm. Because of their larger size, these pollen grains are restrained in the nose and primarily cause AR. Pollen allergens become biologically active upon dissolution of their outer layers which occurs upon exposure to rain/dew, etc. or upon contact with mucous in mucous membranes such as the nasal mucosa or conjunctive. Another important aspect in this is the relationship that pollen grains have with diesel exhaust particles. Air pollution due to diesel causes changes in pollination seasons and increase in pollination duration. The pollens also bind to the small diesel particles and get activated along with the other active metallic ions causing airway inflammation. The activated pollen grains release multiple allergens which are proteases, glycoproteins, and lipocalins. These, once released, bind to the antigen-presenting cells and trigger the Th2 inflammatory cascade in the nasal epithelium.
- *Animal dander:* Animals, such as cat, dog, and rodents are the most common pets and animals found in and around human surroundings. The antigens of these animals are also primarily inhalant allergens which mainly compromise of the lipocalins and albumins. Among these two molecules, the lipocalins are primarily antigenic while the albumins are responsible for cross-reactivity between species. These antigens are found in the epithelial cells of the animal (dander) and also excreted in the urine, saliva, sweat, and other body secretions.
    * *Cat allergen:* Fel d 1 is the major allergen which is a glycoprotein of size 35–39 kDa. Airborne is the major route of transmission, usually carried by the dander of cat where the particle size is 5–10 µm. The Fel d 1 is a very sticky allergen and very light; hence, it is easily airborne and transmitted to not pet areas on clothing and other vehicles and stays on carpets, curtains, etc. The antigen settles down within 2 days but can also be airborne for up to 2 weeks. The presence of 1 µg/g of dust of Fel d 1 is said to be the sensitizing threshold.
    * *Dog allergen:* Can f 1 is the major allergen and is a lipocalin. Other antigens are Can f 2, Can f 4, Can f 5, and Can f 6. This is also a light

antigen which is easily airborne but not as sticky. It is of a similar size of 5–10 µm. The sensitizing threshold has been 2 µg/g of dust.
- *Rodent allergen:* The major mouse antigen is Mus m 1 which is a light and airborne allergen carried on other particles of size up to 10 µm and can be easily inhaled to cause symptoms.
- *Food allergens:* In many cases, food allergens can also present with symptoms of AR. The intake of the causative food can precipitate symptoms of AR. The causative foods can be any among the major food allergens (milk, egg, and peanut) or any food to which that child/adult is allergic.

Environmental Pollutants

- *Environmental tobacco smoke (ETS):* ETS has been found to have a deleterious effect on the sinonasal epithelium. There is increased production of eotaxin-1 and eosinophil accumulation in the airway epithelium along with reduced ciliary beat frequency and chloride ion transport. These mucosal changes can aggravate the symptoms of AR. Studies done on mice have shown that ETS aggravated symptoms of AR after short-term exposure. Similarly, human studies done also showed the worsening of AR with ETS exposure. An interesting fact that came about was that maternal smoking was directly linked to childhood AR. Among adolescents, studies have shown that novel tobacco products such as e-cigarettes and heated tobacco products have been linked with increasing the risk of AR. In conclusion, ETS acts as an irritant and may not causatively be associated with AR; however, it aggravates the symptoms of AR.
- *Traffic-related air pollutant (TRAP):* TRAP is a complex mixture of gases and suspended particulate matter (PM) produced by motor vehicles. TRAP is a mixture of nitrous oxide and nitrogen oxides, especially nitrogen dioxide, elemental carbon, ultrafine particles, fine particle matter (PM2.5), coarse particle matter (PM10), and carbon dioxide. From the intrauterine period, TRAP exposure has been implicated to affect the airway development. Prenatal and early life are critical periods for lung morphogenesis and maturation, during which exposure to environmental pollutants may lead to structural alterations and altered repair mechanisms that are long-term functional changes of organs, resulting in long-lasting impairment of resistance to infection and increases the risk of allergies later in life. Several epidemiological studies have reported that exposure to TRAP during pregnancy and early life increases the risk of allergy to multiple allergens. In more recent studies, exposure to fine particle matter (PM2.5), black carbon, and nitrogen dioxide

during pregnancy and the first 3 years of life was found to be associated with increased morbidity of AR. A positive association between PM2.5 absorbance and the incidence of AR was also described in this study.
- *Smoke exposure:* Exposure to other smoke containing PM has been known to aggravate the symptoms of AR. The sources of this smoke are primarily causes of indoor/household air pollution—incense sticks, air fresheners, mosquito repellents, and vaporizers.

■ PATHOPHYSIOLOGY

The allergic inflammation is primarily a Th2 response to the above-mentioned allergens. The main cellular component is the mast cell and the response is the type 1 hypersensitivity reaction. The reaction has two components:
1. The initial sensitization phase **(Flowchart 1)**
2. The response phase **(Flowchart 2)**

Mast Cells and Mediators

The mast cells are found in maximum concentration beneath the nasal epithelium near the nasal capillaries, near the sensory nerves, and near the glands in the nasal mucosa. The degranulation then produces the nasal congestion, the sneezing and the watery rhinorrhea respectively accompanied

Flowchart 1: Sensitization phase.

```
The allergen is first exposed to the nasal mucosa and is identified by
the antigen-presenting cells (APCs)
                    ↓
APCs engulf the allergen and break the antigen into peptides with the cell
                    ↓
These peptides are then bound to the class II MHC molecules and presented on
the cell surface to the CD4+ T lymphocytes
                    ↓
The activated T lymphocytes then produce IL4, IL5, IL9, and IL13 as well as
expresses CD40L on its cell surface
                    ↓
This causes the CD40 on the B lymphocyte to bind to the CD40L and triggers the IgE
production by the B cells
                    ↓
These IgE antibodies now bind to the high-affinity receptors on the mast cells and
basophils
```

(IgE: immunoglobulin E; IL4: interleukin 4; MHC: major histocompatibility complex)

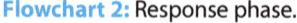

Flowchart 2: Response phase.

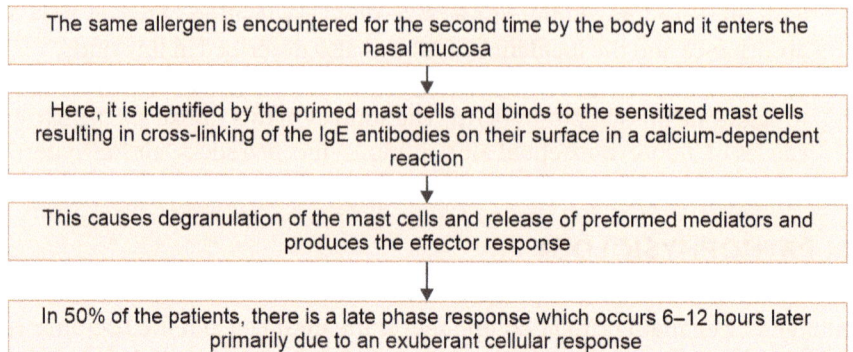

by nasal itching. These are brought about initially by preformed mediators and the reaction is sustained by the sized mediators which are produced by other inflammatory cells such as basophils and eosinophils.

Preformed mediators: These are already formed and stored in granules. They are histamine, serotonin, protease enzymes, and chemotactic factors (eosinophil and neutrophil chemotactic factor). The main preformed mediator produced by the mast cell is histamine. It causes all the initial reactions at the time of mast cell degranulation, i.e., sneezing, nasal congestion, nasal itching, and watery nasal discharge.

Synthesized mediators: These are formed after activation of the cells and breakdown of membrane phospholipids at degranulation. The release is slower, and the effects hence appear later at nearly 6 hours after the initial reaction; however, the reaction is sustained and this is what produces the airway epithelial changes over a period of time. The mediators are leukotrienes (LTC4, LTD4, and LTE4, and LTB4), prostaglandin D2 (PGD2), platelet-activating factor, bradykinins, and cytokines such as TNFα, IL3, and IL5.

Other Cells in Allergic Inflammation

Cellular response involves basophils, eosinophils, and in a lesser number of neutrophils. Out of these, eosinophils play a major role and tissue eosinophilia is very characteristic of AR. The eosinophils cause nasal epithelial desquamation, hyperresponsiveness, and subepithelial fibrosis by causing release of free oxygen radicals, eosinophil cationic protein, and peroxidases. Mast cells and basophils also secrete mediators which help in eosinophil survival and chemotaxis.

Following the release of eosinophilic mediators in the nasal mucosa, there is also chemokine release, such as RANTES, eotaxin, and monocyte chemotactic protein. These chemokines cause increased production of nitric oxide in the nasal epithelium by inducing nitric oxide synthase in mast cells, neutrophils, and eosinophils. Nitric oxide is a potent vasodilator and produces the nasal congestion and mucosal changes in the nasal mucosa.

Role of Neurotransmitters

As the nose is rich with sensory nerve fibers, allergic inflammation also affects the nerves and causes release of neurotransmitters. One of the novel neurotransmitters is substance P which causes increase in vascular permeability. This neurotransmitter also causes elicitation of reaction in nasal provocation tests.

These changes occur throughout the nasal mucosa including the paranasal sinuses and result in epithelial denudation, extracellular matrix deposition, and basement membrane disruption.

■ SUMMARY

Allergic rhinitis manifests in genetically predisposed individuals once they encounter responsible allergens in the environment. Airborne route is the most common trigger factor with common allergens, and agents which are responsible are house dust mites, cockroaches, animal danders, pollens, and spores. After a complex immune interaction, a series of mediators (mostly with mast cell degranulation) is released causing typical symptoms.

■ KEY POINTS

- It is a complex interaction of genes and environmental factors which result in manifestations of AR in an individual.
- Environmental pollutants can be nonspecific trigger which can enhance clinical reactions in an allergic individual by nonimmunological mechanisms.
- A deep understanding of pathophysiology is necessary for effective management of AR in stepwise manner.

■ SUGGESTED READING

1. Chen T, Norback D, Deng Q, Huang C, Qian H, Zhang X, et al. Maternal exposure to PM(2.5)/BC during pregnancy predisposes children to allergic rhinitis which varies by regions and exclusive breastfeeding. Environ Int. 2022;165:107315.
2. Choi BY, Han M, Kwak JW, Kim TH. Genetics and Epigenetics in Allergic Rhinitis. Genes (Basel). 2021;12(12):2004.
3. Chung SJ, Kim BK, Oh JH, Shim JS, Chang YS, Cho SH, et al. Novel tobacco products including electronic cigarette and heated tobacco products increase risk of allergic rhinitis and asthma in adolescents: analysis of Korean youth survey. Allergy. 2020;75:1640-8.

4. Lin SY, Reh DD, Clipp S, Irani L, Navas-Acien A. Allergic rhinitis and secondhand smoke: a population based study. Am J Rhinol Allergy. 2011;25:66-71.
5. London NR Jr, Lina I, Ramanathan M Jr. Aeroallergens, air pollutants, and chronic rhinitis and rhinosinusitis. World J Otorhinolaryngol Head Neck Surg. 2018;4(3):209-15.
6. Ober C, Yao TC. The genetics of asthma and allergic disease: A 21st century perspective. Immunol. Rev. 2011;242:10-30.
7. Ramasamy A, Curjuric I, Coin LJ, Kumar A, McArdle WL, Imboden M, et al. A genome-wide meta-analysis of genetic variants associated with allergic rhinitis and grass sensitization and their interaction with birth order. J Allergy Clin Immunol. 2011;128:996-1005.
8. Sbihi H, Allen RW, Becker A, Brook JR, Mandhane P, Scott JA, et al. Perinatal Exposure to Traffic-Related Air Pollution and Atopy at 1 Year of Age in a Multi-Center Canadian Birth Cohort Study. Environ Health Perspect. 2015;123(9):902-8.
9. Singh S, Sharma BB, Salvi S, Chhatwal J, Jain KC, Kumar L, et al. Allergic rhinitis, rhinoconjunctivitis, and eczema: prevalence and associated factors in children. Clin Respir J. 2018;12:547-56.
10. Suojalehto H, Lindstrom I, Majuri ML, Mitts C, Karjalainen J, Wolff H, et al. Altered microRNA expression of nasal mucosa in long-term asthma and allergic rhinitis. Int Arch Allergy Immunol. 2014;163:168-78.
11. Van Beijsterveldt CE, Boomsma DI. Genetics of parentally reported asthma, eczema and rhinitis in 5-yr-old twins. Eur Respir J. 2007;29:516-21.
12. Waage J, Standl M, Curtin JA, Jessen LE, Thorsen J, Tian C, et al. Genome-wide association and HLA fine-mapping studies identify risk loci and genetic pathways underlying allergic rhinitis. Nat Genet. 2018;50:1072-80.

CHAPTER 4

Allergic Rhinitis: Comorbidities

Swati Kalra

■ INTRODUCTION

Allergic rhinitis (AR) is a systemic allergic disease which poses a huge burden of rhinitis in childhood and adolescence. In pediatric population, almost 8% children between 6 and 8 years are affected with AR and its prevalence increases up to 35% in adolescents. AR does not occur in isolation rather it coexists with several other comorbid conditions. About 75% of children with AR develop other concomitant conditions including conjunctivitis, asthma, atopic dermatitis (AD), rhinosinusitis, otitis media with effusion (OME), or adenoid hypertrophy (AH). Apart from these, AR also impairs the quality of life (QoL) due to sleep disorders and obstructive sleep apnea. Therefore, it appears more to be a part of a systemic disease rather than being a separate entity alone. Association of AR with other comorbidities has been hypothesized to be caused by systemic inflammatory response affecting both the upper and lower airways as a part of united airway concept.

The comorbidities associated with AR can be subdivided into various subgroups depending upon their origin. First subgroup includes those diseases which are part of spectrum of allergic diseases, e.g., asthma, AD, food allergy, and anaphylaxis. Second group includes those disorders which are anatomically related to the nose, such as conjunctivitis, sinusitis, middle ear problems, throat, and laryngeal effects. Third category includes problems related to sleep, behavior, and QoL. Identification and management of other comorbidities are important for improving the overall QoL of patients with AR.

■ ASTHMA

Asthma represents a chronic inflammatory disorder of lower airways affecting all age groups including children and adolescents. It has been addressed as a serious public health concern globally. Common features of asthma include inflammatory changes in small airways, typically characterized by bronchial inflammation which increases after exposure to certain triggers, such as allergens, irritants, or infections.

Allergic rhinitis and asthma are recognized as often seen together for the simple reason that these two are distinct clinical manifestations of underlying immunoglobulin E (IgE)-mediated inflammatory disease affecting the respiratory tract. The allergic symptoms of the upper and lower airways can be regarded as manifestations of a shared atopic condition, and AR and asthma are often treated as a unified concept. The high comorbidity between AR and asthma is well-established, with approximately 10–40% of individuals with AR also experiencing asthma, while over 80% of asthmatics also have AR. AR serves as a risk factor for the development of asthma, and its diagnosis often precedes the onset of asthma. Both adults and pediatric age groups have demonstrated an increased risk of asthma among individuals with AR, with childhood AR specifically elevating the risk of asthma development in preadolescence and adolescence age groups. The risk of asthma increases more in patients with perennial AR compared to seasonal AR and maximum risk being seen in children sensitive to house dust mite. Various clinical investigations also reveal the increased sensitivity of bronchial mucosa in patients with AR, more so during pollen season. Hence, both perennial as well seasonal AR have increased risk of manifesting as asthma.

Assessing the presence of asthma in patients with moderate-to-severe AR is essential due to the interconnected nature of these conditions. Poorly controlled AR can exacerbate asthma, leading to increased healthcare visits due to bronchial symptom exacerbations.

It has been observed that AR patients also have lower airway hyper-responsiveness. Various mechanisms have been proposed to explain the link between AR and asthma including nasal dysfunction, the nasobronchial reflex, rhinovirus adhesion theory, and the migration of T cell responses. Nasal dysfunction interferes with humidification, filtration, and sterilization of inhaled air. Nasobronchial reflex is a reflex in which stimulation of upper airway mucosa causes bronchoconstriction of lower airway by vagal and trigeminal pathways; hence, worsening asthma symptoms. Apart from these mechanisms, various inflammatory compounds produced in upper airways are aspirated as well as absorbed into blood stream, hence, leading to bronchoconstriction in the lower airways. Furthermore, recent evidence suggests that small airway respiratory dysfunction precedes the development of asthma in children with AR, indicating it to be a potential early marker for asthma progression.

Understanding the intricate relationship between AR and asthma is crucial for effective management and treatment strategies. Recent studies have shed light on various aspects of this relationship, highlighting the importance of comprehensive care for individuals affected by both conditions.

■ OBESITY

Obesity has been emerging as a worldwide pandemic disease affecting all age groups. It has been found to have associations with many human diseases including cancers, allergies, and diseases of immunological system. There are evidences to suggest an association between AR and obesity in terms of increased body mass index (BMI) more so in the pediatric population. Obesity is a lifestyle disorder caused mainly due to physical inactivity and changing trends in the modern lifestyle. The changes have documented ill effect on immune system, leading to reduced tolerance to antigens. Dysregulation of immune system links it to predisposition to allergic diseases. This dysregulation happens due to various mechanisms. Obese individuals have a relatively proinflammatory state due to increased expression of interleukin-1β (IL-1β) and elevated levels of leptins which change the functioning of the immune system as well. Increased levels of leptin upregulate the expression of type 2 innate lymphoid cells (ILC2s) which have been proposed to be involved in AR development. This makes the symptoms of allergies worse and last longer. Another mechanism of immune dysregulation leading to allergic disorders is linked to eosinophils. Eosinophils are the primary effector cells responsible for ongoing airway inflammation leading to allergic disorders. They have also been recognized to play a role as proinflammatory cells aggravating the symptoms in AR, asthma, and AD. Higher leptin levels have been found to be associated with increased eosinophil activity at the site of inflammation. Therefore, obesity serves as a predisposing condition for AR. In therapy, BMI reduction is effective as it leads to a reduction in inflammation and stabilization of the course of AR.

■ QUALITY OF LIFE

Although AR is not life-threatening, its impact on QoL is significant, affecting social interactions, self-esteem, and academic performance. This disruption can lead to absenteeism, decreased work productivity, impaired concentration, and learning difficulties, making QoL deterioration a key indicator of disease severity. Nasal obstruction, a predominant symptom of AR, profoundly impacts QoL. The symptoms of pediatric AR often disrupt sleep, resulting in fatigue, daytime sleepiness, and irritability. Sleep disturbances in turn result in memory impairment, depression, and behavioral disturbances. Children with AR may exhibit shyness, depression, anxiety, or fearfulness.

Adolescents with AR experience QoL challenges similar to adults but may have fewer sleep disturbances and more difficulties with concentration, particularly related to schoolwork. Although they may not report as much interference with daily activities or emotional disturbances as adults but the scholastic performance is definitely hampered. Assessing the impact of AR on QoL is facilitated by the use of generic and specific questionnaires, such as the Rhinoconjunctivitis Quality of Life Questionnaire (RQLQ), including its pediatric (PRQLQ) and adolescent (AdolRQLQ) versions.

Researchers have examined the QoL and symptom profile of patients across different age groups and observed that presence of nasal obstruction and nasal itching have a significant impact on QoL of adolescents and children, highlighting age-related differences in symptom perception. A recent study focused on pediatric patients with persistent allergic rhinitis (PER) revealed that nonresponders to medical treatment reported worse QoL scores compared to responders, with nasal symptoms being particularly impactful in both adolescents and children.

Gender differences in QoL among adolescents have also been noted, with females showing worse QoL scores, possibly reflecting variances in symptom reporting and self-assessment of health. Female gender has been identified as a risk factor for impaired QoL in AR and asthma. Additionally, gender differences in the subjective perception of nasal symptoms have been observed in pediatric patients. These findings underscore the importance of considering gender-specific factors in evaluating and managing QoL in patients with AR.

■ CHRONIC RHINOSINUSITIS

Sinusitis or more commonly known as rhinosinusitis is inflammation of nasal sinuses which occurs following infection or blockage of nasal passages. Chronic rhinosinusitis (CRS) in children is characterized by inflammation of the nasal and paranasal sinus mucosa, necessitating the presence of at least two symptoms, with one being nasal congestion or nasal discharge, enduring for >12 weeks. Additional symptoms may include facial pain, loss of smell, or cough, alongside endoscopic or computed tomography (CT) evidence indicative of sinus involvement.

Sinusitis has been proposed to a predecessor of rhinitis and rarely occurs without concurrent rhinitis. The symptomatology of both acute and CRS often overlaps with those of PER including nasal congestion, rhinorrhea, loss of smell, and cough. This shared symptomatology complicates accurate diagnosis, particularly in settings where nasal endoscopy and CT scans are unavailable.

The relationship between rhinosinusitis and respiratory allergy remains contentious. While AR has been identified as a comorbidity in pediatric CRS, but different studies have found diverging results in this context. Some investigations suggest a higher prevalence of atopy markers in children with CRS, while others have failed to establish AR as a significant risk factor for CRS in allergic children with chronic sinonasal symptoms lasting for >3 months. This discrepancy could be due to variations in defining CRS and AR across studies. Hence, there exists a complexity of the relationship between AR and CRS, necessitating further research for a comprehensive understanding of their interplay.

ADENOID HYPERTROPHY

The adenoid (also known as the nasopharyngeal tonsil) is a part of nasal-associated lymphoid tissue (NALT) complex which is centrally located in the nasopharynx just behind the posterior orifice of nasal apertures. Many-a-times, repeated exposure to allergens and infections of upper airways results in proliferation of NALT, leading to an increase in the volume of the adenoid tissue and blockage of nasopharyngeal airway. Since nose and adenoids are in close proximity to each other, the presence of local allergic inflammation, including the synthesis of total and specific IgE results in hypertrophy of lymphoid cell populations of adenoids as well in children with AR.

Review of literature has shown variable results in context to correlation between AR and AH. While few studies suggest that the prevalence of AH is more in allergic children compared to nonallergic children with the average prevalence of AH being 5–6%. Furthermore, the presence of positive allergic tests for aeroallergens has been strongly associated with AH. The pathogenesis of co-occurrence of AR and AH has been hypothesized to be due to presence of allergic/eosinophilic inflammation occurring in adenoids of children with AR. Patients who have AH are more likely to have persistent rhinitis for prolonged duration and the predominant symptom is nasal congestion. While those without AH have runny nose as the predominant symptom.

Recent research has further explored the impact of AH on the severity and duration of AR and the results reveal that children with AH have a higher prevalence of PER. Not only prevalence, but severity of illness also increases in children who have co-occurrence of AH and AR. Hence, PER and AH may go hand in hand with AR manifesting as recurrent disease and complicating the management of AH by increasing resistance to treatment.

ALLERGIC CONJUNCTIVITIS

Allergic conjunctivitis is a clinical manifestation of allergic disorders affecting eyes. It is characterized by intense eye itching, conjunctival hyperemia/injection, chemosis, and watering eyes. It is one of the most common comorbidities associated with AR, and for this reason, it is also referred to as allergic rhinoconjunctivitis. Approximately 33–56% of cases of allergic conjunctivitis coexist with AR, likely due to mutual anatomical connections between the nasal mucosa and the ocular surface. The prevalence and severity of conjunctival symptoms associated with AR vary with several factors. As per literature review, allergic conjunctivitis symptoms occur more often in patients with seasonal AR compared to perennial AR. About 75% of patients with seasonal AR have co-occurrence of conjunctivitis. Skin prick tests of these patients show sensitization to seasonal pollens more than house dust mite. Itching of the ears and throat can also be associated with AR.

ATOPIC DERMATITIS

Atopic dermatitis is one of the most common chronic inflammatory disorders according to World Health Organization (WHO) affecting millions of people worldwide. It has been postulated to be the first step toward the development of the atopic march beginning in first year of life. It poses a huge socioeconomic burden in the developed nations and off late in developing countries as well. Currently, about 15 and 20% of the children and between 1 and 10% of the adult population have been found to be affected by AD. Studies from various birth cohorts have shown that AD is frequently observed to co-occur with AR in children. Among the diseases of allergic spectrum, AR has been found to be the most prevalent atopic disease alongside AD. Coexistence of AR and AD has been associated with aeroallergen sensitizations namely of house dust mite, cockroach, and feather-specific allergens, whereas those with AD alone have elevated rates of wheat, peanut, and soybean-specific IgE.

The effects of this co-occurrence are multifaceted. While some data suggest that a greater extent of allergic disease leads to more severe reactions, others indicate an inverse relationship between exacerbations in skin and respiratory symptoms. Notably, in patients presenting with asthma, AD, and AR, systemic glucocorticoid bioavailability poses a significant concern, as treatment often targets multiple sites including the skin, bronchi, and nasal passages. Treatment modalities of both AR and AD include allergen avoidance, saline douching, antihistamines, antileukotrienes, immunotherapy, and anticytokines. Management of one also improves the outcome of other as treatment modalities often overlap. However, there is a need to find the exact association between these conditions.

OTITIS MEDIA WITH EFFUSION

Atopy and AR are the predisposing factors for OME, as there is evidence to suggest that treating allergies may alleviate otological symptoms. Older children with AR are at a greater risk of developing OME compared to younger ones; hence, necessitating the treatment of AR to stop their progression into OME. Proposed mechanisms linking AR and OME include allergic inflammation within the respiratory epithelium of the Eustachian tube, potentially leading to tubal dysfunction. Additionally, allergic responses involving the middle ear mucosa support the concept of a united airway.

SUMMARY

Allergic rhinitis is a systemic allergic disease posing a huge burden in childhood and adolescence. Association of AR with comorbidities increases the morbidity and found to be associated by the same inflammatory response as a part of unified airway concept. The most common comorbidities are asthma, obesity, conjunctivitis, and chronic rhinosinusitis. Adequate management of comorbidities is also essential for management of AR and improve quality of life.

■ KEY POINTS

- Allergic rhinitis has an increased prevalence and there are unmet needs to alleviate certain issues associated with the same.
- Children and adolescents with AR presenting with comorbidities have a significant impact on their QoL.
- AR comorbidities also confer increased health and socioeconomic burden on AR patients.
- Management of comorbidities is very important for improving treatment outcomes of AR.

■ SUGGESTED READING

1. Ibanez MD, Valero AL, Montoro J, Jauregui I, Ferrer M, Davila I, et al. Analysis of comorbidities and therapeutic approach for allergic rhinitis in a pediatric population in Spain. Pediatr Allergy Immunol. 2013;24(7):678-84.
2. Iordache A, Balica NC, Horhat ID, Morar R, Tischer AA, Milcu AI, et al. A Review Regarding the Connections between Allergic Rhinitis and Asthma—Epidemiology, Diagnosis and Treatment. Curr Health Sci J. 2023;49(1):5-18.
3. Knudgaard MH, Andreasen TH, Ravnborg N, Bieber T, Silverberg JI, Egeberg A, et al. Rhinitis prevalence and association with atopic dermatitis: A systematic review and meta-analysis. Ann Allergy Asthma Immunol. 2021;127(1):49-56.e1.
4. Mariño-Sánchez F, Valls-Mateus M, de Los Santos G, Plaza AM, Cobeta I, Mullol J. Multimorbidities of Pediatric Allergic Rhinitis. Curr Allergy Asthma Rep. 2019;19(2):13.
5. Mariño-Sánchez F, Valls-Mateus M, de Los Santos G, Plaza AM, Cobeta I, Mullol J. Multimorbidities of Pediatric Allergic Rhinitis. Curr Allergy Asthma Rep. 2019;19(2):13.
6. Roberts G, Xatzipsalti M, Borrego LM, Custovic A, Halken S, Hellings PW, et al. Paediatric rhinitis: position paper of the European academy of allergy and clinical immunology. Allergy. 2013;68:1102-16.
7. Scadding GK. Rhinitis and Sinusitis. Clin Res Med. 2008:409-23.
8. Yücel Ekici N, Külahci Ö. Relationship between tissue and serum eosinophilia in children undergoing adenotonsillectomy with allergic rhinitis. Turk J Med Sci. 2019;49(6):1754-9.
9. Zhang X, Sun B, Li S, Jin H, Zhong N, Zeng G. Local atopy is more relevant than serum sIgE in reflecting allergy in childhood adenotonsillar hypertrophy. Pediatr Allergy Immunol. 2013;24(5): 422-6.

SECTION 2
Diagnostics

Section Editor: Gayatri S Pandit

- **Clinical Diagnosis: Rhinitis and Comorbidities**
  Dinesh Naik

- **Structural Assessment**
  Veena Singh Gupta

- **Functional Assessment**
  Swikaar H Panchal

- **Inflammatory Assessment in Allergic Rhinitis**
  Antarbhai Patel

- **Allergy Tests**
  *Taha A Qureshi, Tabasum Shafi, Ayaz Gull,
  Aabid M Koul, Muzima Jeelani, Roohi Rasool*

Clinical Diagnosis: Rhinitis and Comorbidities

Dinesh Naik

■ INTRODUCTION

Diagnosis of rhinitis may appear obvious from the chief complaints, but a detailed, accurate history and a complete thorough examination is required for better phenotyping of rhinitis. Understanding the triggers, family history, comorbid conditions, and response to earlier treatment helps in better and holistic management.

A detailed history not only helps in diagnosis but also aids in selecting allergens for allergy testing and correlations of the results of the tests.

History could be taken in following headings, presenting complaints, past history, treatment history, socioeconomic history, family and personal history, and clinical review of systems.

The presenting complaints include:
- Nasal congestion
- Sneezing
- Itching
- Rhinorrhea
- Postnasal drip
- Conjunctival irritation

■ NASAL CONGESTION

Nasal congestion can make toddlers struggle to breath with sniffing and snorting or may have sneezing, elder ones tend to repeatedly blow their nose. More the exposure to the allergen, greater and severe are the symptoms. Nasal congestion tends to be more severe in the night, causing snoring and leading to breathing through the mouth. Sometimes, it is so severe that not only sleep is disturbed but children may have apnea episodes and wake up with a gasp. Also lack of proper sleep can lead to tiredness, easy fatigability, daytime somnolence, headache, increased irritability, and even cognitive impairment. It is imperative to know that normally the nose gets blocked on one side for some time followed by spontaneously opening but closure of other side which is called nasal cycle or nasal pulse. Also, it is known that the nose can get blocked on the side, one is turning while sleeping (dependent side). Nasal septal deviation and hypertrophied inferior turbinate can commonly cause persistent unilateral nasal congestion; some other causes could be nasal polyp, foreign body (especially with foul smell and fairly recent history), or rarely, even a tumor.

SNEEZING

Allergic rhinitis is often marked by outbursts of 5–10 sneezes. Sneezing is often noticed in the morning hours. Early morning sneezing is found to be typical of house dust mite allergy.

ITCHING

Besides itching of nose, patient may also complaint itching of eyes, oral mucosa, and face and itchy ears. Nasal pruritus and sneezing are hallmark of histamine-mediated response.

RHINORRHEA

Rhinorrhea or nasal discharge is usually clear to little opaque liquid and bilateral. Thick yellowish purulent secretions are usually seen in chronic sinusitis or atrophic rhinitis. Unilateral clear rhinorrhea could be due to cerebrospinal fluid (CSF) leak.

POSTNASAL DRIP

Postnasal drip is one of the most common characteristics of chronic rhinitis, and over a prolonged period of time, it may lead to a chronic sore throat, a chronic cough, or recurrent throat clearing.

CONJUNCTIVAL IRRITATION

The eyes symptoms include itching, redness, and watering, which probably arise, in part, from a naso-ocular reflex besides allergic response to direct exposure of eyes to the same allergen and are found in 50% of allergic rhinitis cases. Presence of atopic conjunctivitis determines choice of treatment.

When other symptoms such as cough, headache, altered smell, and bad breath are present, check for any coexistent conditions which will alter the treatment decision.

SEASONALITY OF SYMPTOMS

Perennial symptoms are quite often because of house dust mites, cockroach allergens, and few molds. Seasonal symptoms usually indicate an outdoor allergen as a potential culprit. Differentiating into seasonal and perennial allergic rhinitis may be tricky at times as seasonal allergens may vary from year to year, in some countries pollens may be present for up to 10 months per year. Conversely, patients' exposure to perennial factors may be intermittent, for example, with only occasional contact with domestic pets. Also many patients may be allergic to multiple allergens; so the seasonal symptoms to each allergen will lead to prolonged duration of the symptoms, presenting as persistent nasal complaints. As human travel has become more accessible and affordable, they get exposed to different aeroallergens leading to unique pattern of symptoms including the severity and the duration. Hence, understanding migration history of patient is also relevant here.

■ DIURNAL VARIATION

Rhinitis symptoms worsen during the early morning hours due to circadian variations in inflammation. House dust mite allergy typically presents as morning symptom. Pollen-related allergy tends to get better as day progresses.

■ LOCATION OF SYMPTOMS

Indoor allergens such as house dust mite, animal dander, cockroach, or mold trigger symptoms at home, whereas pollens are more responsible for symptoms in outdoor environment.

■ FAMILY HISTORY

Allergic rhinitis is known to have strong genetic component. Having a first-degree relative with atopic allergic conditions it increases the risk of suffering from allergic symptoms. If either mother or father is affected, the chance of child having atopy is 30–50%, and risk increases to 60–80%, if both parents are affected. There is 25–35% risk in the presence of an atopic sibling. 12% of children with allergic rhinitis have no family history of allergic rhinitis suggesting other etiological factors.

■ ENVIRONMENTAL HISTORY

The patient's home *environment details* should be sought to identify any potential triggers as it is crucial in establishing a clinical correlation. If symptoms arise promptly on exposure to allergen, it suggests immunoglobulin E (IgE)-mediated allergy. Dust mites are commonly found in warm, humid areas, and on curtains, beds, mattresses, and carpets. Child sleeping with soft toys or favorite blankets is also prone to exposure to dust mites. Mold mainly grows in damp environment, over walls containing water pipes, and around air-conditioner vents.

Environmental history of school or place at work is also very important to know. Exposure to occupational allergens or irritants, such as perfumes, gases, dough, sawdust, plastic, and animal products can be responsible for the allergic symptoms. Also, if symptoms occur only during work or immediately after work or only at workplace and if one is free of symptoms during weekends or holidays, it may strongly indicate allergen exposure at work. A person's exposure to allergens may also depend on where he spends lot of his time, such as for studies, sports, gym, or any other activity; so this history also is pertinent toward the diagnosis.

■ NONALLERGIC TRIGGERS

Sometimes, other *triggers* may be responsible for allergy-like symptoms (nonallergic rhinitis), namely the airborne substances considered as irritants, including volatile organic compounds such as detergents, paints, perfumes, fumes and particulate air pollutants, such as smoke, fumes, and gases released on burning fuel. Weather changes and climatic conditions, such as sudden change of temperature, water vapor content, or different altitude are also contributing factors in nonallergic rhinitis.

■ DRUG HISTORY

A thorough recent *drug history* is mandatory as some drugs, such as β-blockers, nonsteroidal anti-inflammatory drugs (NSAIDs), salicylates, angiotensin-converting enzyme (ACE) inhibitors, and certain hormones can lead to symptoms of rhinitis. Also assessing patient response to over-the-counter antihistamines and intranasal steroids may help in diagnosis of allergic rhinitis and creating proper management plan. Any history of being on alternative medicine should be noted **(Table 1)**.

TABLE 1: Medications associated with chronic nasal symptoms.

Antihypertensives	Angiotensin-converting enzyme inhibitors
	β-adrenergic blockers
	Amiloride
	Prazosin
	Hydralazine
Psychotropics	Risperidone
	Chlorpromazine
	Amitriptyline
Phosphodiesterase-5 inhibitors	Sildenafil
	Tadalafil
	Vardenafil
Nonsteroidal anti-inflammatory drugs	Ibuprofen
Others	Gabapentin

Source: Adkinson NF Jr, Bochner BS, Burks AW, Busse WW, Holgate ST, Lemanske RF Jr, et al. Middleton's Allergy: Principles and Practice, 8th edition. Philadelphia, PA: Elsevier/Saunders; 2013. p. 670.

Consistent, reproducible symptoms associated with particular allergen or trigger and symptom-free period in the absence of exposure help in establishing a potential trigger.

■ COMORBIDITIES

Any patient suffering from one allergic disease has high chances of having another allergic disease, such as allergic rhinoconjunctivitis, acute and chronic sinusitis, nasal polyps, acute and chronic otitis media, asthma, food allergy, drug allergy, and atopic dermatitis. According to Bousquet J et al. 2001, around 40% of patients with chronic rhinitis have asthma, and 80% of patients with asthma have allergic rhinitis like symptoms. Fokkens et al. 2007 found that allergic rhinitis was noted in 30% of patients with acute sinusitis, 67% with unilateral chronic sinusitis, and 80% with bilateral chronic sinusitis **(Fig. 1)**.

Child with respiratory allergies may frequently also have food allergy, which is considered a risk factor for other allergic diseases. The concept of atopic march states that usually infants who have food allergy and atopic dermatitis in infancy may develop asthma and allergic rhinitis in later life but it is found commonly that it may not follow any particular order rather all allergic conditions come under one umbrella of atopic diseases. Goksör et al. concluded in his study that 40% of children with history of food allergies in

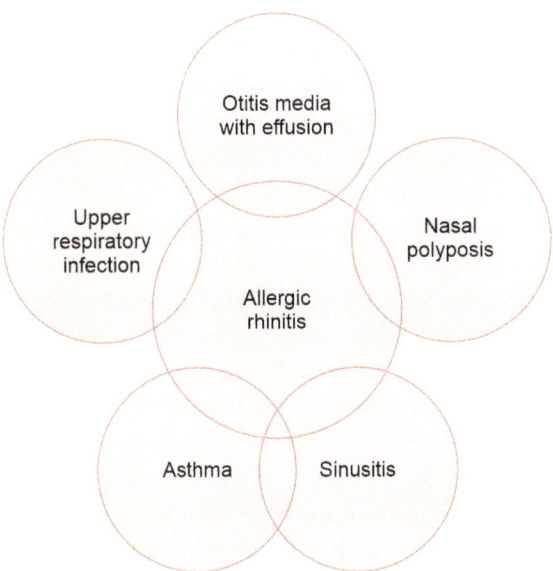

Fig. 1: Allergies coexist.
Source: Spector SL. Overview of comorbid associations of allergic rhinitis. J Allergy Clin Immunol. 1997;99(2):S773-80.

infancy developed allergic rhinitis by 8 years of age. Allergic rhinitis, asthma, and eczema are 2–4 times more common in children with food allergies. One study showed that 77.4% of children with food allergies developed rhinitis or asthma by 7 years of age compared to 45.5% without food allergies.

Rhinitis may also be one of several manifestations of true food allergy. Food allergies can trigger allergic symptoms in the nose, eyes, or throat along with gastrointestinal symptoms but respiratory allergies are usually <6%. Eating hot and spicy foods can cause watering of eyes and running nose. Also, certain foods may directly stimulate the autonomic nervous system leading to rhinitis like symptoms. This is called gustatory rhinitis. It is nonimmunological in origin.

In some cases, when one is sensitized to some allergens may develop oral symptoms on eating food with similar structural allergen. This is called *oral allergy syndrome*. It is a separate and distinct IgE-mediated syndrome. For example, patient sensitized to an Inhalant allergen Birch pollen can have oral/pharyngeal itching and swelling after the ingestion of certain foods, especially apples, hazelnuts, and stone fruits. In a study, 17% of the patients with pollen allergy developed allergic reaction to some fruits and vegetables. It is a manifestation of cross-reactivity between inhaled allergens and certain heat-labile ingested proteins. Similar symptoms are seen on eating seafood such as shrimps and crabs in dust mite allergic patients.

Sleep disorders are commonly seen in allergic rhinitis with severe nasal obstruction present as lack of quality sleep, repeated arousals from sleep, apneas leading to daytime drowsiness, and other symptoms. Also migraines are commonly seen in allergic rhinitis patients.

The patients with chronic problem may also lose their sense of smell and taste. Onset of hyposmia/anosmia indicates polypoidal changes around middle turbinate and hence demands endoscopic examination. Many allergic rhinitis patients may develop otitis media with effusion (OME) and also it is noted that atopic children have more incidence of bilateral OME with more noticeable hearing loss comparatively. Hence in persistent or recurrent OME, any associated allergic rhinitis should be identified and treated.

It is important to ask about the effects of allergic rhinitis on the patient's quality of life, school, or work absenteeism, without which complete and accurate assessment of clinical picture is not possible.

Allergic Rhinitis and its Impact on Asthma (ARIA) group reclassified allergic rhinitis (2001) as "Intermittent" (symptoms <4 days per week or <4 weeks per year) and "Persistent" (symptoms >4 days per week and >4 weeks per year) category. On the basis of severity of symptoms, such as performance at work or in school, daily activities, and quality of sleep, it was further categorized as "mild" and "moderate-severe" **(Fig. 2)**.

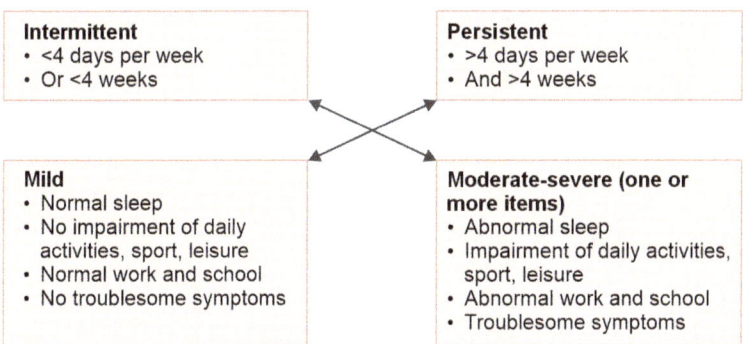

Fig. 2: Classification of allergic rhinitis.
Source: Min YG. The pathophysiology, diagnosis and treatment of allergic rhinitis. Allergy Asthma Immunol Res. 2010;2:65-76; Gupta N. Allergy in a Nutshell, Kindle edition. New Delhi: Jaypee Brothers Medical Publishers (P) Ltd.; 2019. p. 83.

■ PHYSICAL EXAMINATION

The routine physical examination should be done to assess the cause or triggers of rhinitis and gauge the severity of symptoms, as well as identify other comorbidities and complications. The nose need to be primarily examined, but one should also look at the face, eyes, ears, throat, and neck. Chest and dermatological examination also need to be done.

Facial Features

When the nose is itchy and dripping due to allergies, people with allergic rhinitis tend to wipe or rub their nose upward with an open palm or fingers to relieve the itching or the blockage. This often becomes habitual gesture and is called *allergic salute* **(Figs. 3A and B)**. It leads to upward tilting of the tip of the nose and creating a prominent transverse fold of skin over the bridge of the nose called *nasal crease*. Other signs include facial dysmorphism, dental crowding, and malocclusion of jaw. The continuous mouth breathing gives a distinct appearance to face which is often referred to as *allergic gape* **(Fig. 4)**. Prolonged nasal congestion leads to venous stasis under the eyes leading to dark boggy appearance below the eyes which is called *allergic shiners* **(Fig. 5)**.

Nose

Examine the nasal cavity with a nasal speculum or some may use an otoscope with nasal adapter. If experienced and trained, flexible rhinolaryngoscope may be used to evaluate nasal septum, turbinate, middle meatal area, and nasopharynx.

The nasal mucosa over the turbinates is usually swollen with a pale, bluish-gray color in allergic rhinitis, whereas in nonallergic rhinitis cases, it

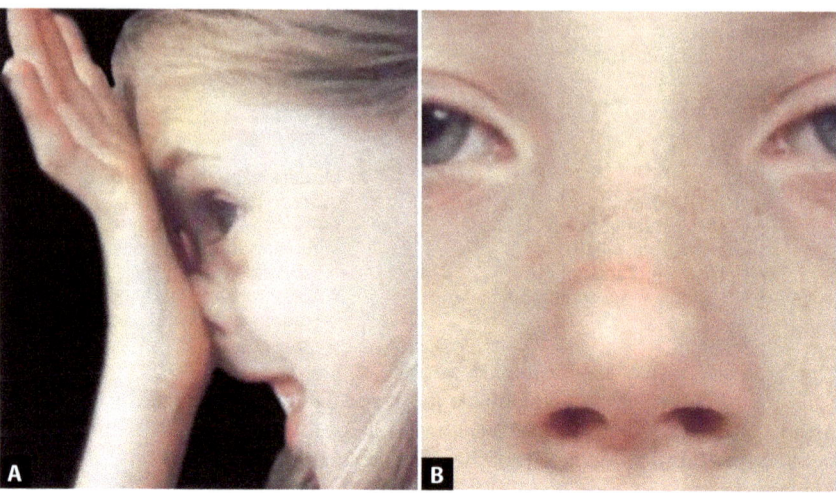

Figs. 3A and B: Allergic salute and nasal crease.
Source: [online] Available from https://qph.cf2.quoracdn.net/main-qimg-14afe257e1f6a3f75f6c21bd33fd1e99-lq [Last accessed July, 2024].

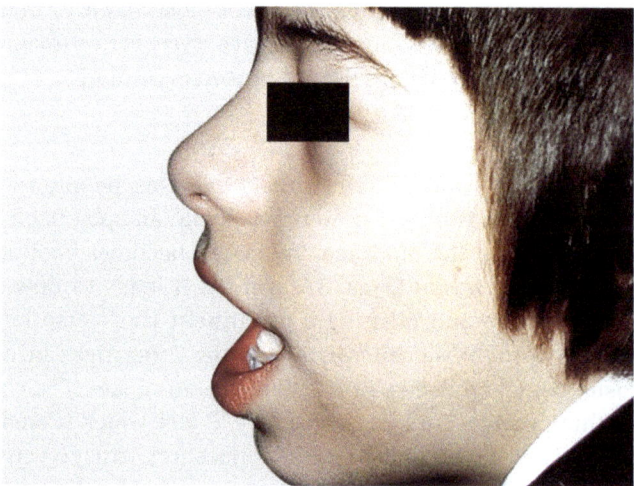

Fig. 4: Allergic gape.
Source: [online] Available from https://obgynkey.com/wp-content/uploads/2016/07/B9780323079327000053_f004-016-9780323079327.jpg [Last accessed July, 2024].

is pink or erythematous but these changes cannot differentiate between both the entities **(Figs. 6A and B)**.

Note the consistency and amount of nasal mucus. Thin and clear watery secretions are usually seen in allergic rhinitis, while white or thick yellow secretions are common with sinusitis. Crusting may indicate atrophic rhinitis.

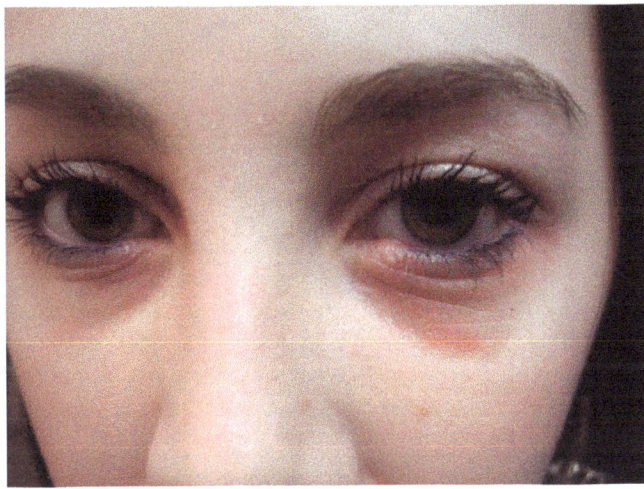

Fig. 5: Allergic shiners.
Source: [online] Available from https://upload.wikimedia.org/wikipedia/commons/thumb/b/b6/Allergic_shiner_in_pediatric_patient.png/440px-Allergic_shiner_in_pediatric_patient.png [Last accessed July, 2024].

Examine the nasal septum for any deviation or perforation, which is seen in chronic or atrophic rhinitis, certain granulomatous disease, topical decongestant, or steroid misuse.

Examine the nasal cavity for polyps, foreign body, or tumors. Polyps are gray masses hanging by a stalk, which can be differentiated from turbinate by their gray, shiny grape-like and cystic appearance **(Fig. 7)**. Also, topical decongestant shrinks the turbinates but not the polyps. Polyps are insensitive to touch unlike the turbinates. One can probe around the polyps whereas turbinates are attached to lateral wall **(Table 2)**.

Ears, Eyes, and Oropharynx

Examine the tympanic membrane with the otoscope. Normal tympanic membrane will appear pearly white with shiny cone of light. Look for abnormalities such as retraction of the tympanic membrane, air bubbles, or fluid levels which is seen in dysfunction of eustachian tube or otitis media secondary to allergic rhinitis. Also look for tympanic membrane mobility with pneumatic otoscopy.

Eyes may show erythema and swelling of the conjunctivae, with excessive watering. Do not miss the Dennie-Morgan lines which are the creases seen below the lower eyelid **(Fig. 8)**.

Check the throat for tonsillar enlargement and "cobblestoning"—bulgings in the posterior pharynx mucosa due to enlargement lymphoid tissue on the

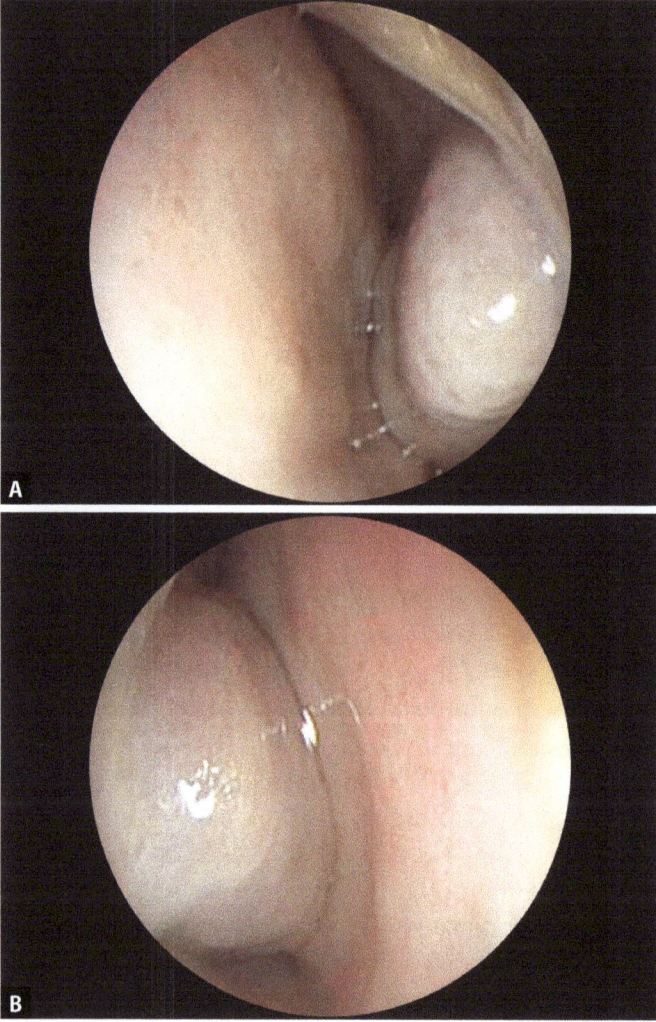

Figs. 6A and B: Endoscopic image of nasal cavity in allergic rhinitis. Pale and boggy nasal mucosa is seen in a case of allergic rhinitis. The nasal airway is blocked as inferior turbinates touch the nasal septum bilaterally left (A) and right (B) nasal cavity.
Source: [online] Available from https://doctorlib.info/pediatric/pediatric-otorhinolaryngology-diagnosis-treatment/pediatric-otorhinolaryngology-diagnosis-treatment.files/image030.jpg [Last accessed July, 2024].

posterior pharynx. Notice any malocclusion or a high-arched palate as it is commonly seen in mouth breathers **(Fig. 9)**.

Neck

Palpate the neck for lymph nodes or examine the thyroid gland.

CHAPTER 5: Clinical Diagnosis: Rhinitis and Comorbidities

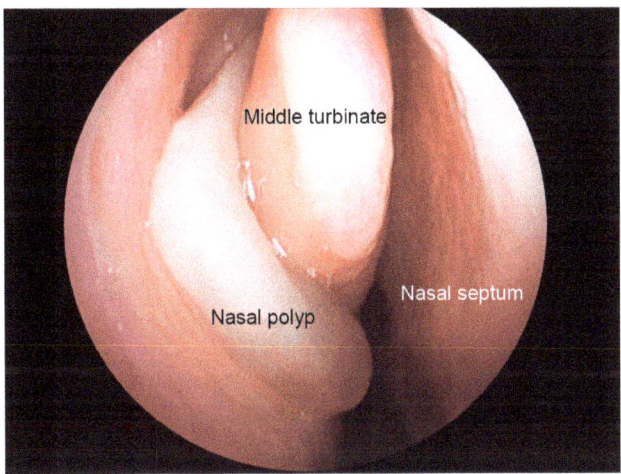

Fig. 7: Nasal polyp.
Source: [online] Available from https://b35-2508914.smushcdn.com/2508914/wp-content/uploads/2021/08/image019.png?lossy=1&strip=1&webp=1 [Last accessed July, 2024].

TABLE 2: Pattern of rhinitis.

Feature	Seasonal allergic	Perennial allergic	Nonallergic
Symptoms	Rhinorrhea, sneezing, itchy nose, watery and itchy eyes	Rhinorrhea, sneezing, itchy nose, watery and itchy eyes	Nasal blockage and postnasal drainage prominent
Other atopic diseases	Common	Common	Less common
Age of onset	Most before 20 years	Most before 20 years	Over 20 years
Timings	During affected seasons only	Throughout the year	Perennial, can coexist with allergic rhinitis
Triggers	Grass cutting, windy weather, walking out of house, walking through parks, gardening	Vacuuming, dry dusting, pet exposure, opening old cupboards	• No readily identifiable aeroallergens • *Respiratory irritants:* Cigarette smoking, strong scents, fragrances • *Weather changes:* Temperature, humidity • *Others:* Spicy foods, medications, infections
Likely allergens	Grass, weed, tree, pollens	House dust mite, cats, dogs, fungus	None

Source: Gupta N. Allergy in a Nutshell, Kindle edition. New Delhi: Jaypee Brothers Medical Publishers (P) Ltd.; 2019. p. 83.

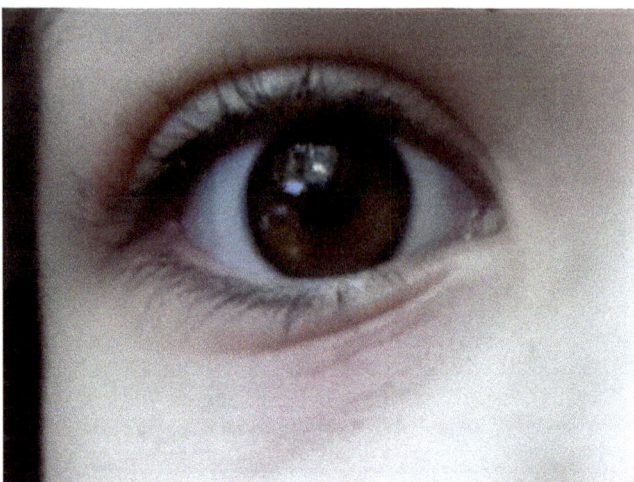

Fig. 8: Dennie–Morgan lines.
Source: [online] Available from https://upload.wikimedia.org/wikipedia/commons/8/83/Dennie-Morgan-Falte.jpg [Last accessed July, 2024].

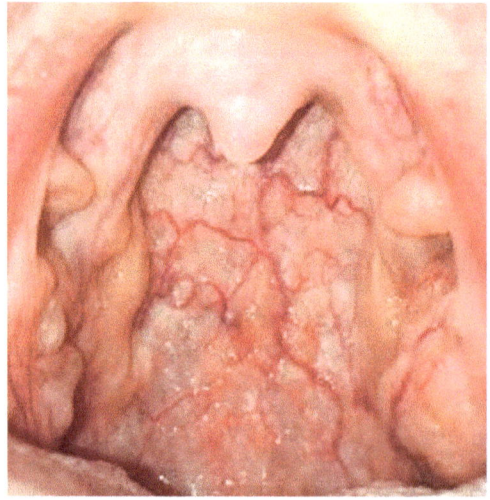

Fig. 9: Cobblestone appearance of pharynx.
Source: [online] Available from https://qph.cf2.quoracdn.net/main-qimg-049d80380c58589c8c126483c29e8d96-lq [Last accessed July, 2024].

Chest

Examine the chest for wheezing, crackles, pronged expiratory phase, use of accessory muscles, hyperinflation, and rubs.

SYSTEMIC EXAMINATION

Search for any signs of systemic diseases which also have nasal symptoms, such as cystic fibrosis, immunodeficiency, primary ciliary dyskinesia, thyroid disorders, rheumatic disorders, examination of skin, cardiovascular system, and abdomen and central nervous system (CNS) should be part of systemic examination **(Flowchart 1)**.

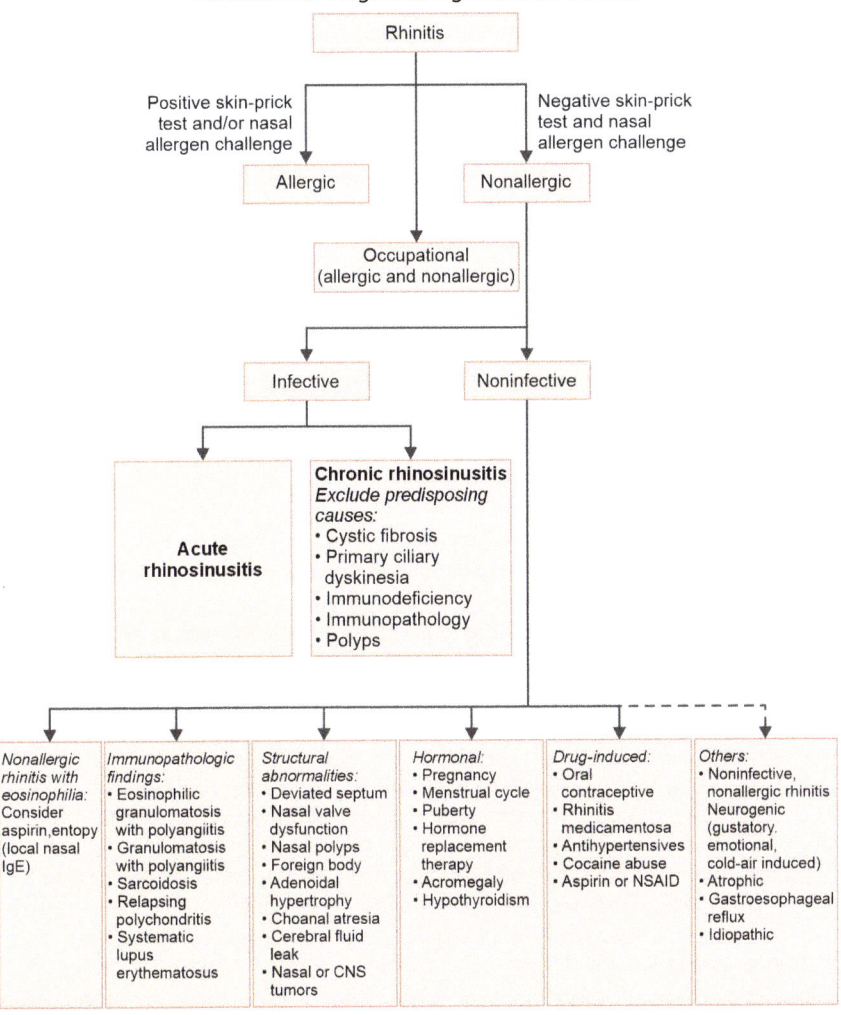

Flowchart 1: Diagnostic algorithm for rhinitis.

(CNS: central nervous system; IgE: immunoglobulin E; NSAID: nonsteroidal anti-inflammatory drug)
Source: Adapted from Greiner AN, Hellings PW, Rotiroti G, Scadding GK. Allergic rhinitis. Lancet. 2011;378(9809):2112-22.

■ SUMMARY

History taking and physical examination help the clinician to diagnose allergic rhinitis, differentiate between allergic and nonallergic rhinitis, categorize it and thus guide in the formulation of treatment strategy and plan.

■ KEY POINTS

- Allergic rhinitis is the diagnosis based on history. Therefore, history taking is pivotal in the management.
- The typical spectrum of symptoms in allergic rhinitis includes nasal blockage and itching, sneezing, nasal discharge, postnasal drip and conjunctival redness, and itching.
- History should include detailing of environmental history, drug history, social history, and family history as well as seasonality, location of symptoms, triggering factors, and response to earlier medications.
- Examination should not only aid in diagnosis of allergic rhinitis but also should aim at identifying comorbidities.

■ SUGGESTED READING

1. Adkinson NF, Bochner BS, Busse WW, Holgate ST, Lemanske R, Simons FER. Middleton's Allergy: Principles and Practice, 7th edition. Philadelphia: Mosby Elsevier; 2009.
2. Adkinson NF Jr, Bochner BS, Burks AW, Busse WW, Holgate ST, Lemanske RF Jr, et al. Middleton's Allergy: Principles and Practice, 8th edition. Philadelphia, PA: Elsevier/Saunders; 2013. pp. 1-1764.
3. Baroody FM, Foster KA, Markaryan A, deTineo M, Naclerio RM. Nasal ocular reflexes and eye symptoms in patients with allergic rhinitis. Ann Allergy Asthma Immunol. 2008;100(3):194-9.
4. Bousquet J, Van Cauwenberge P, Khaltaev N; Aria Workshop Group; World Health Organization. Allergic rhinitis and its impact on asthma. J Allergy Clin Immunol. 2001;108(5 Suppl):S147-334.
5. Eccles R. A role for the nasal cycle in respiratory defence. Eur Respir J. 1996;9:371-6.
6. Fokkens W, Lund V, Mullol J; European Position Paper on Rhinosinusitis and Nasal Polyps group. European position paper on rhinosinusitis and nasal polyps 2007. Rhinol Suppl. 2007;20:1-136.
7. Fornadley JA, Corey JP, Osguthorpe JD, Powell JP, Emanuel IA, Boyles JH, et al. Allergic rhinitis: clinical practice guideline. Committee on Practice Standards, American Academy of Otolaryngic Allergy. Otolaryngol Head Neck Surg. 1996;115(1):115-22.
8. Goksör E, Loid P, Alm B, Åberg N, Wennergren G. The allergic march comprises the coexistence of related patterns of allergic disease not just the progressive development of one disease. Acta Paediatr. 2016;105(12):1472-9.
9. Hadley JA. Evaluation and management of allergic rhinitis. Med Clin North Am. 1999;83(1):13-25.

10. Jung S, Lee SY, Yoon J, Cho HJ, Kim YH, Suh DI, et al. Risk factors and comorbidities associated with the allergic rhinitis phenotype in children according to the aria classification. Allergy Asthma Immunol Res. 2020 Jan;12(1):72-85.
11. Kjellman NI. Atopic disease in seven-year-old children. Incidence in relation to family history. Acta Paediatr Scand. 1977;66(4):465-71.
12. Kliegman R, Stanton B, Geme JW, Schor NF, Behrman RE, Nelson WE. Nelson Textbook of Pediatrics, 21st edition. Philadelphia, PA: Elsevier Inc; 2020.
13. Malik V, Ghosh S, Woolford TJ. Rhinitis due to food allergies: fact or fiction? J Laryngol Otol. 2007;121(6):526-9.
14. Martines F, Martinciglio G, Martines E, Bentivegna D. The role of atopy in otitis media with effusion among primary school children: audiological investigation. Eur Arch Otorhinolaryngol. 2010;267(11):1673-8.
15. Muliol J, Maurer M, Bousquet J. Sleep and allergic rhinitis. J Investig Allergol Clin Immunol. 2008;18(6):415-9.
16. Ownby DR. Environmental factors versus genetic determinants of childhood inhalants allergies. J Allergy Clin Immunol. 1990;86:279-87.
17. Singh K, Axelrod S, Bielory L. The epidemiology of ocular and nasal allergy in the United States, 1988-1994. J Allergy Clin Immunol. 2010;126:778-83.
18. Small P, Keith PK, Kim H. Allergic rhinitis. Allergy Asthma Clin Immunol. 2018;14(Suppl 2):51.
19. Tewfik TL, Mazer B. The links between allergy and otitis media with effusion. Curr Opin Otolaryngol Head Neck Surg. 2006;14(3):187-90.
20. Tsai JD, Chang SN, Mou CH, Sung FC, Lue KH. Association between atopic diseases and attention-deficit/hyperactivity disorder in childhood: a population-based case-control study. Ann Epidemiol. 2013;23(4):185-8.
21. Vedanthan PK, Nelson H. Allergy skin testing. In: Vedanthan PK, Nelson HS, Agashe SN, Mahesh PA, Katial R (Eds). Textbook of Allergy for the Clinician. Boca Raton, Florida: CRC Press; 2021.
22. Vázquez-Nava F, Quezada-Castillo JA, Oviedo-Treviño S, Saldivar-González AH, Sánchez-Nuncio HR, Beltrán-Guzmán FJ, et al. Association between allergic rhinitis, bottle feeding, non-nutritive sucking habits, and malocclusion in the primary dentition. Arch Dis Child. 2006;91(10):836-40.
23. Weider DJ, Baker GL, Salvatoriello FW. Dental malocclusion and upper airway obstruction, an otolaryngologist's perspective. Int J Pediatr Otorhinolaryngol. 2003;67:323-31.
24. Zeiger RS, Heller S. The development and prediction of atopy in high-risk children: follow-up at age seven years in a prospective randomized study of combined maternal and infant food allergen avoidance. J Allergy Clin Immunol. 1995;95(6):1179-90.

CHAPTER 6

Structural Assessment

Veena Singh Gupta

■ INTRODUCTION

Diagnosis of allergic rhinitis is made on clinical grounds. It is based on the presence of four cardinal symptoms which include: (1) watery rhinorrhea, (2) sneezing, (3) nasal obstruction, and (4) nasal pruritus. This is often associated with itching eyes, nose, and palate and can lead to secondary symptoms, such as fatigue, irritability, somnolence, and postnasal discharge.

Severity is mostly determined by Allergic Rhinitis and its Impact on Asthma (ARIA) guidelines depending on the number of days or weeks a symptom is present and its effect on lifestyle, e.g., sleep, daily activities, sport, leisure, school and work, and presence of troublesome symptoms.

Although the diagnosis can be made clinically, a thorough examination of the nose and associated structures for comorbidities can help confirm the diagnosis, ascertain severity of disease and its complications, and also rule out causes of nonallergic rhinitis.

Assessment modalities for structural analysis of allergic rhinitis include:
- Rhinoscopy—anterior and posterior
- Otoendoscopy
- X-ray
- Computed tomography (CT) scan nose and paranasal sinus (PNS)
- Magnetic resonance imaging (MRI)

■ STRUCTURAL EXAMINATION

Anterior Rhinoscopy

No examination of the nose is complete without a per speculum examination with a nasal speculum (e.g., Vienna, Thudicum, and Killian) and headlight. In every young child, anterior nasal examination can be done by just lifting the tip of the nose **(Fig. 1)**.

Structures to be observed in anterior rhinoscopy are as follows:
- *Nasal passages:* They are narrow in septal deviation or with hypertrophied turbinates and wider in atrophic rhinitis.
- Septum—for position, spurs, deviation, color of mucosa, crusting, perforations, and any abscesses or swellings.
- Floor of the nose—for any defects (cleft or fistula), swelling, e.g., cysts and granulations.

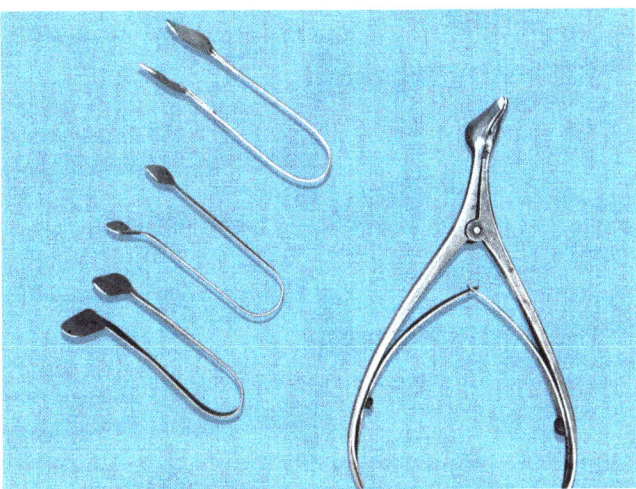

Fig.1: Nasal Thudicum and Vienna speculum.
Courtesy: N C Jindal Institute of Medical Sciences, Hisar, Haryana.

- Roof—only seen in case of atrophic rhinitis.
- Nasal mucosa—color, secretions, crusting, etc.
- Inferior turbinate and the tip of the middle turbinate can be seen easily.
- Any visible polyps.

Normal sinus mucosa is pink on examination. Patients with allergic rhinitis mostly have a clear serous discharge. Swelling of turbinates can be seen with a pale or bluish appearing mucosa. Some types of nonallergic rhinitis can also have pale or erythematous mucosa. Dry, crusting mucosa can be seen in atrophic rhinitis. Watch for any discharge/polyp in the inferior/middle meatus. Look for localized congestion in case of suspected sinusitis.

Nasal Endoscopy

Major drawback of anterior rhinoscopy is that it can evaluate only anterior two-thirds of the nasal cavity, and hence, large part of nasal cavity remains unexamined. Hence, nasal endoscopy examination is important in specific cases **(Fig. 2)**.

Usually, nasal endoscopy is extension of routine anterior nasal examination. Allergologists may consider nasal endoscopy in specific cases of allergic rhinitis.

Indications for nasal endoscopy in allergic rhinitis may include but not be limited to the following:
- Initial assessment of patients experiencing symptoms suggestive of sinusitis such as nasal obstruction or congestion or mucopurulent drainage, facial pain or pressure, or anosmia

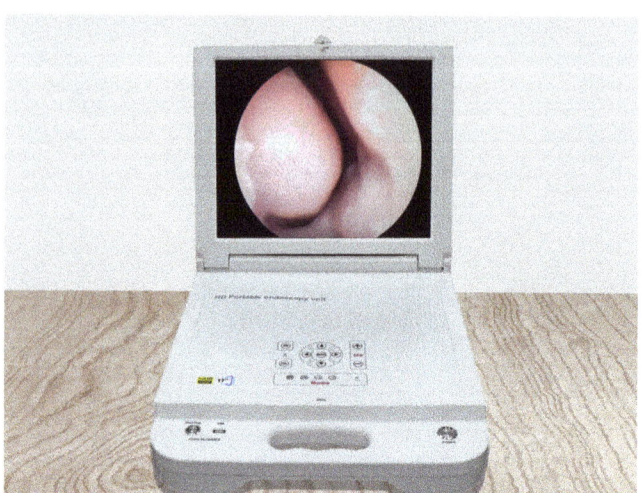

Fig. 2: Right inferior turbinate hypertrophy.
Courtesy: N C Jindal Institute of Medical Sciences, Hisar, Haryana.

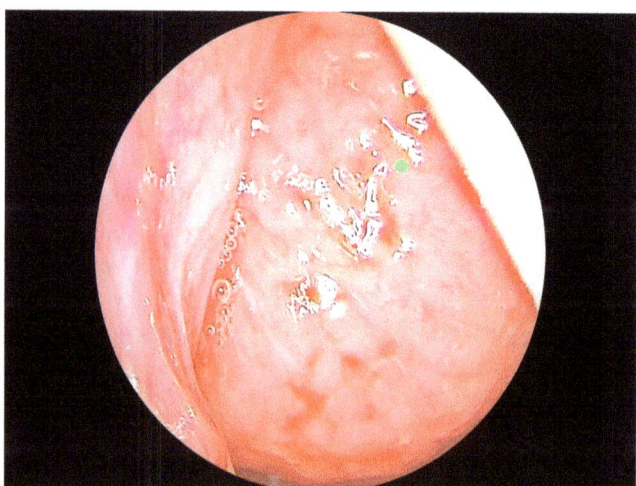

Fig. 3: Grade 4 adenoid hypertrophy in nasopharynx.
Courtesy: N C Jindal Institute of Medical Sciences, Hisar, Haryana.

- Evaluation of complications of rhinosinusitis
- Evaluation of patients response to medical treatment (e.g., resolution of polyps, secretions, and mucosal edema after treatment)
- Unilateral nasal or sinus disease suggesting foreign bodies, polyps, or tumors **(Fig. 3)**
- Surgical procedures if and when required, e.g., debridement and removal of crusting from obstructed nasal and sinus cavities.

Diagnostic nasal endoscopy can be done with either flexible or rigid endoscope. Endoscope used is 0° and 2 mm pediatric scope.

Preparation

Nasal cavity is decongested with gauze soaked with xylometazoline and 4% xylocaine for topical anesthetic action 5 minutes before endoscope. Pediatric scopes are very small and in an experienced hand preparations may not be even required.

Various study results have documented a >90% correlation between endoscopically obtained cultures and maxillary sinus aspirates, making endoscopically-guided cultures the current criterion standard.

Scope is passed in three times:
1. In the *first pass*, the scope is passed along the floor of the nasal cavity and into the nasopharynx with the patients head in flexion. First seen are the inferior meatus and opening of the nasolacrimal duct. The scope is then advanced posteriorly to examine the nasopharynx along with openings of the eustachian tube and the fossa of Rosenmüller.
2. In the *second pass*, the endoscope is passed between the middle and inferior turbinates to examine the inferior portion of the middle meatus, the sphenoethmoid recess, the slit-like or oval ostia of the sphenoid sinus, and the superior turbinate. While withdrawing, rotate laterally to see the infundibulum, uncinate, and ethmoid bulla.
3. The *third pass* often requires a 30º endoscope or head repositioning to see the olfactory cleft area.

Otoscopy

Same endoscope or an otoscope can be used for the quick examination of the tympanic membrane. Normal appearance of tympanic membrane is described as pearly white/gray with cone of light in anteroinferior quadrant with movements of drum to be noted with Valsalva. Look for any abnormalities such as retraction or fullness of the ear drum, fluid behind ear drum, or diminished mobility of the eardrum.

■ X-RAY FOR THE NASAL CAVITY AND PARANASAL SINUSES

A number of radiographic views are available to view the sinuses. However, the most common are occipitomental (Waters), occipitofrontal (Caldwell), and lateral views **(Fig. 4)**.

Plain radiography is a useful initial assessment for the sinuses being cheap, easily available, and has low radiation dose. But, it is now considered obsolete for the accurate evaluation of sinusitis. However in primary care

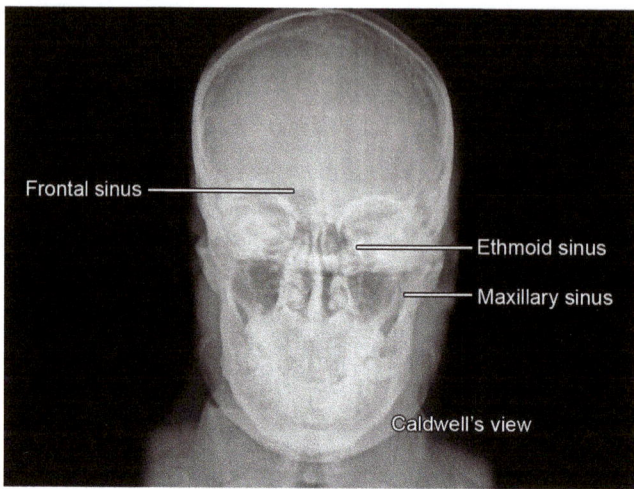

Fig. 4: Caldwell's (occipitofrontal) view depicting the sinuses.
Courtesy: N C Jindal Institute of Medical Sciences, Hisar, Haryana.

and resource depleted settings, it remains an important investigation in the management of sinusitis.

Digital *Caldwell's* view is also called the nose forehead position as the nose and forehead touch the film and the X-ray film is projected from a caudal angle of 15–20°. Caldwell view is very useful for the assessment of frontal and ethmoidal sinus opacification, as well as for nasal septum deviation. However, it provides some limitations in assessment of frontal or ethmoidal mucosal thickening.

Digital *Waters view* is also called the nose chin view as nose and chin touch the film and X-ray beam is projected from the occipital side. It is a reliable modality for maxillary sinus evaluation. Open mouth view can also show the sphenoid sinus. This is the most commonly used view for evaluation for sinusitis **(Fig. 5)**.

In a study, assessing the diagnostic value of Waters radiograph versus CT (as gold standard) for evaluation of 40 patients with sinusitis the sensitivity, specificity, and positive predictive value (PPV) of Waters view was found to be 83.3%, 69.2%, and 83.3%, respectively.

■ X-RAY FOR ADENOIDS

Evaluation of adenoids becomes important part of assessment of allergic rhinitis, especially in pediatric population. Gold standard for adenoid evaluation is nasal endoscopy, however, younger children may not cooperate for endoscopy and X-ray nasopharynx remains as alternative choice in that case.

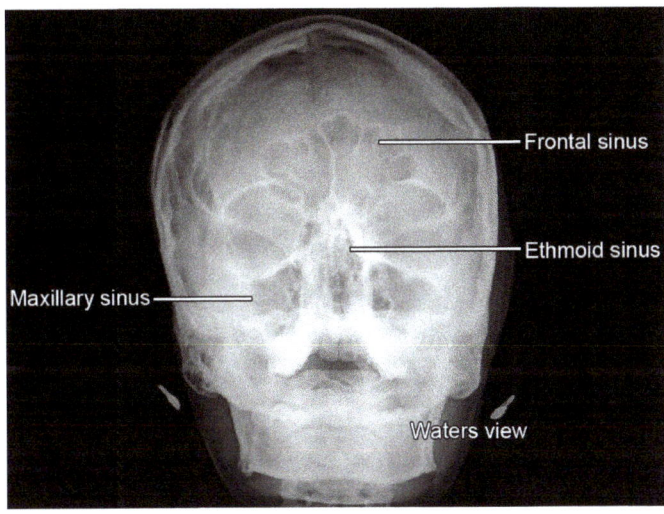

Fig. 5: Waters view for the sinuses.
Courtesy: N C Jindal Institute of Medical Sciences, Hisar, Haryana.

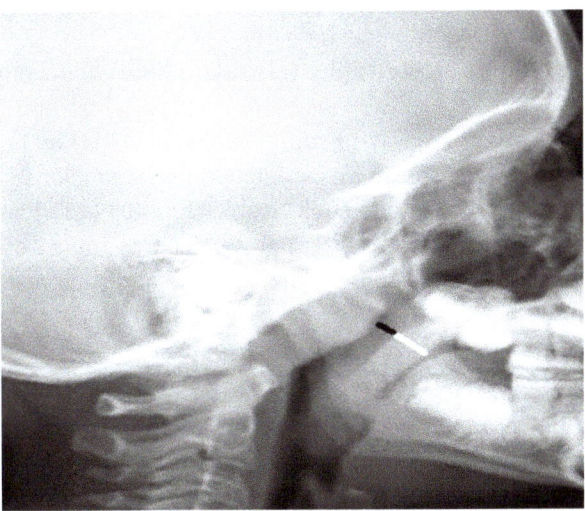

Fig. 6: Adenoidal hypertrophy with airway (black)-to-soft-palate (white) ratio.
Courtesy: N C Jindal Institute of Medical Sciences, Hisar, Haryana.

Cohen and Konak classified adenoidal hypertrophy based on X-ray findings.

While assessing the airway-to-soft-palate ratio, the width of the airway immediately behind the soft palate and the width of the soft palate 1 cm below the hard palate are taken into account **(Fig. 6)**.

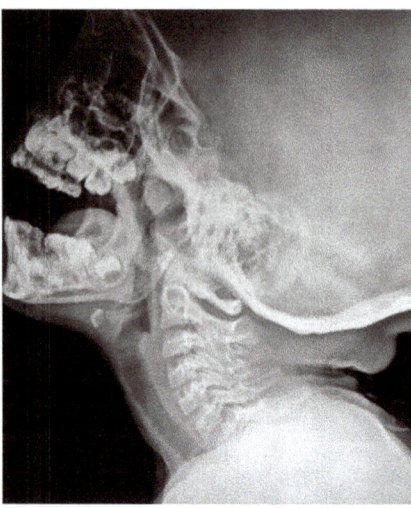

Fig. 7: Lateral soft tissue X-ray of the neck showing moderate adenoidal hypertrophy (AH).
Courtesy: N C Jindal Institute of Medical Sciences, Hisar, Haryana.

Patients are then classified as having:
- Normal (airway-to-soft-palate ratio ≥1)
- Mild-to-moderate hypertrophy (airway-to-soft-palate ratio between 0.5 and 1)
- Severe hypertrophy (airway-to-soft-palate ratio <0.5) **(Fig. 7)**.

Numerous studies have shown an association between allergic rhinitis and adenoidal hypertrophy. In one such study, 90 of 404 (22%) children with allergic rhinitis had adenoidal hypertrophy which was grade 2 or higher.

However, these figures can be highly variable and such results have not been replicated.

■ CONTRAST-ENHANCED COMPUTED TOMOGRAPHY

Imaging studies are usually not needed in allergic rhinitis unless one is suspecting sinusitis or other complications, for which a CT scan is the examination of choice. Coronal CT imaging is the preferred initial procedure and a noncontrast scan usually suffices in most cases **(Figs. 8 and 9)**.

In acute sinusitis, CT scan nose and PNS are ordered only if any complications as suspected whereas in chronic rhinosinusitis (both with polyps and without polyps), it is part of the evaluation **(Figs. 8 to 12)**.

The *CT paranasal sinus protocol* is used as it provides a good means for assessing the mucosa and bone system of the sinonasal cavities. CT provides for excellent resolution and display of soft-tissue attenuation. It can be used to look for any air-fluid levels and polypoid masses within the normally air-filled cavities of the sinuses and nasal cavity. Mucoceles can be formed as a

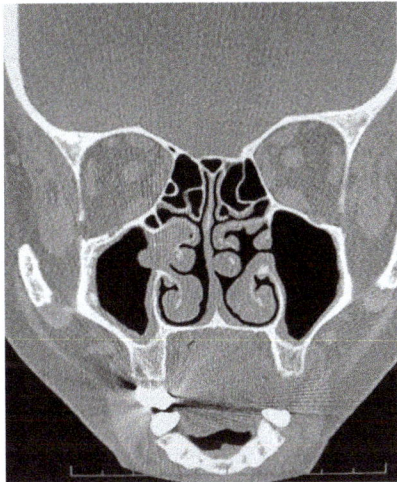

Fig. 8: Bilateral maxillary sinusitis with hypertrophied turbinates and nasal mucosa prolapsing into right maxillary sinus.
Courtesy: N C Jindal Institute of Medical Sciences, Hisar, Haryana.

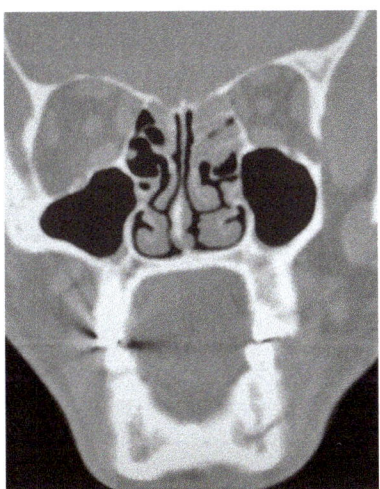

Fig. 9: Bilateral ethmoid and maxillary sinusitis and hypertrophied turbinates.
Courtesy: N C Jindal Institute of Medical Sciences, Hisar, Haryana.

result of obstruction of the sinus ostia in chronic rhinosinusitis and can be visualized as a homogenously opacified sinus cavity with attenuation value similar to mucoid secretion and devoid of air. Also, CT can be used to look for any disease extending beyond the bony perimeters of the sinuses into the adjacent soft tissue of the orbit, brain, and infratemporal fossa.

Typical indications of CT include acute rhinosinusitis, mucoceles, fungal infection, chronic sinusitis, air fluid levels on PNS X-ray, nasal polyposis,

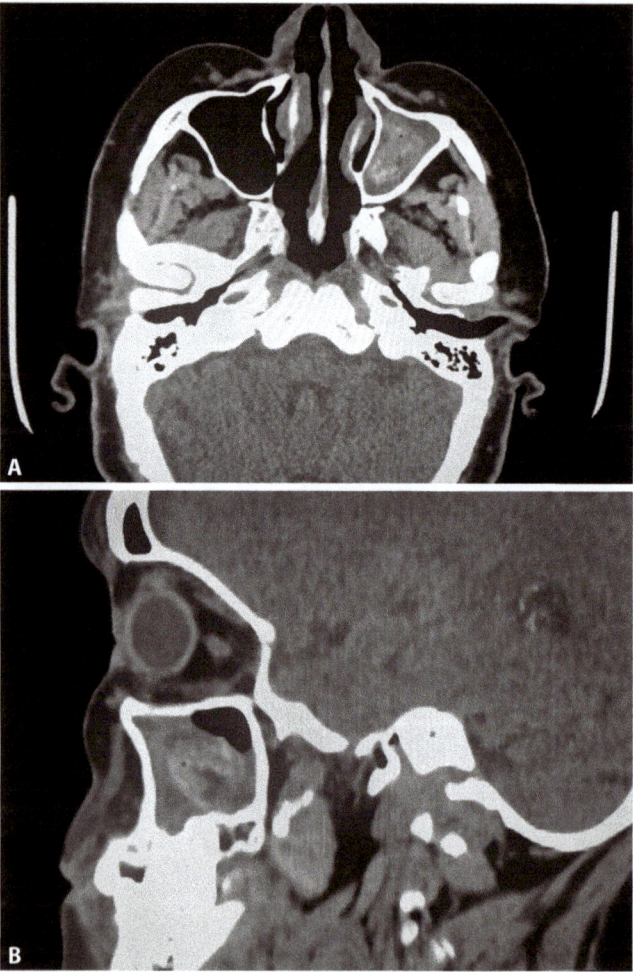

Figs. 10A and B: Left maxillary sinusitis with heterogeneous opacification suggestive of chronic inspissated secretions and/or fungal infection (axial and sagittal views) on CT.
Courtesy: N C Jindal Institute of Medical Sciences, Hisar, Haryana.

facial pressure headache unresponsive to medical treatment, preoperative for sinus surgery, and anosmia **(Fig. 12)**.

CT of the sinuses with contrast is usually done for complications of sinusitis, e.g., subperiosteal abscess and periorbital edema. This helps to differentiate soft-tissue opacification.

■ MAGNETIC RESONANCE IMAGING FOR THE SINUSES

MRI is better than CT in assessing mucosal changes and anomalies because of better soft tissue contrast resolution and tissue characterization.

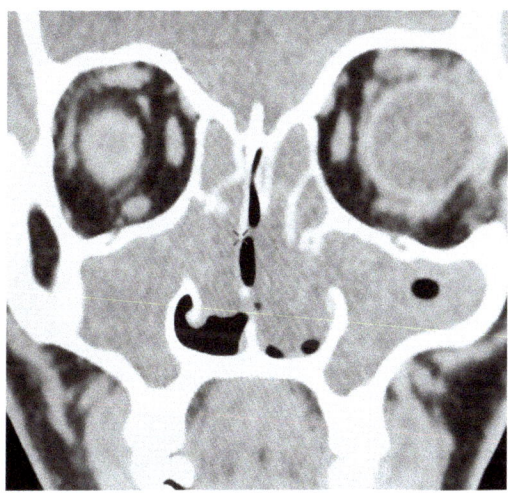

Fig. 11: Pansinusitis with polypoidal mucosal thickening with opacification of bilateral maxillary, frontal, and ethmoid sinuses with hypertrophy of nasal turbinates. Hyperdense areas suggestive of chronic inspissated secretions/fungal infection.
Courtesy: N C Jindal Institute of Medical Sciences, Hisar, Haryana.

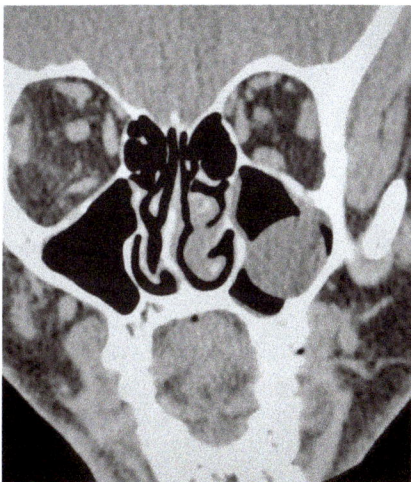

Fig. 12: Left maxillary sinusitis with large polyp; hypertrophied turbinates on the left side with septal deviation.
Courtesy: N C Jindal Institute of Medical Sciences, Hisar, Haryana.

Magnetic resonance imaging is reserved for the evaluation of:
- Complications of local sinus infections, particularly suspected intracranial extensions.
- Orbital involvement.

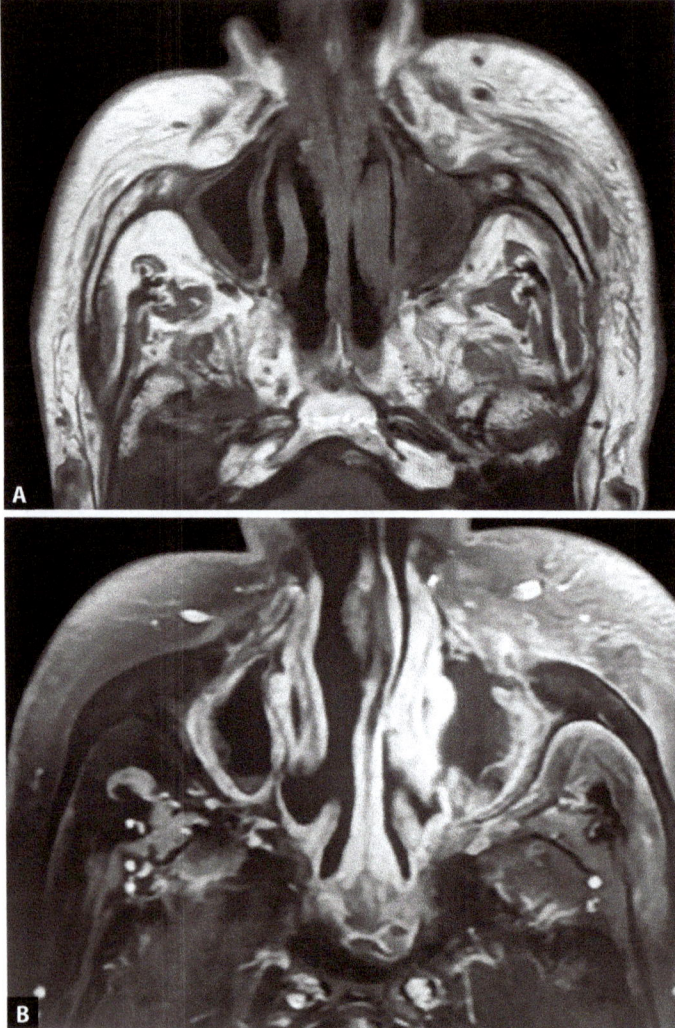

Figs. 13A and B: Maxillary sinusitis on magnetic resonance imaging (MRI) (contrast and noncontrast respectively).
Courtesy: N C Jindal Institute of Medical Sciences, Hisar, Haryana.

- Chronic invasive allergic fungal rhinosinusitis.
- Sinonasal squamous cell carcinomas and other biopsy proven tumors.
- Unilateral sinonasal opacification on CT.

Normal mucosa of the paranasal sinuses appear hyperintense on T2-weighted images. However, CT can help to assess the bony structures better than MRI, and therefore, CT remains the preferred modality for preoperative assessment of patients with chronic sinusitis **(Figs. 13 to 15)**.

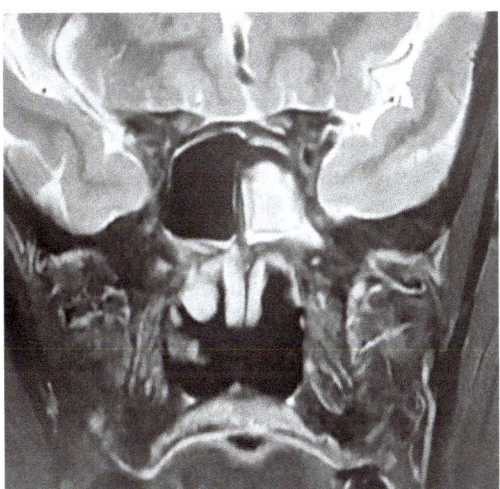

Fig. 14: Sphenoid sinusitis on magnetic resonance imaging (MRI).
Courtesy: N C Jindal Institute of Medical Sciences, Hisar, Haryana.

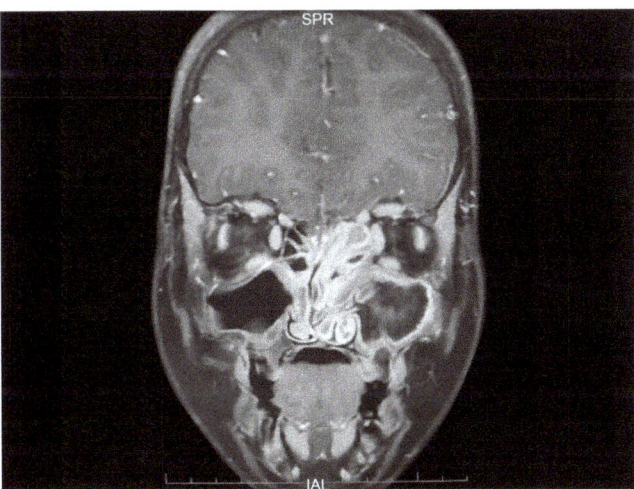

Fig. 15: Polypoidal lesion extending from left maxillary antrum into left nasal cavity via infundibulum. Nasal septum deviated to right. Left maxillary, ethmoid, sphenoid, and bilateral frontal sinuses opacified by nonenhancing chronic inspissated secretions with superimposed fungal infection.
Courtesy: N C Jindal Institute of Medical Sciences, Hisar, Haryana.

SUMMARY

Structural examination of the nose helps to assess severity of disease, complications and associated comorbidities, and anatomical variations in allergic rhinosinusitis.

■ KEY POINTS

- Diagnosis of allergic rhinitis is clinical. However, a good structural assessment is needed to assess severity and complications of the disease. It can also help assess response to therapy and rule out comorbidities.
- A per speculum examination is a good initial assessment for structural changes in allergic rhinitis in the outpatient department (OPD) setting and nasal endoscopy can be done when predominant obstructive symptoms are present.
- X-ray nose and PNS gives incomplete information of sinus.
- CT scan is the diagnostic modality of choice for assessing sinusitis and its complications.
- MRI may be used where complications related to sinus disease are expected.

■ ACKNOWLEDGMENTS

I am grateful to my colleagues at NC Jindal Institute of Medical Sciences for providing clinical pictures for evaluation of allergic rhinitis and thank Dr Madhuri Mehta (HOD and Senior Consultant, Department of ENT, Dr Teenu Singh (Department of Radiology), Dr Mohit Vashishth, and Dr Navroz Mehta (Department of ENT) for their help and cooperation.

■ SUGGESTED READING

1. Byeon H. The association between allergic rhinitis and otitis media: a national representative sample of in South Korean children. Sci Rep. 2019;9:1610.
2. Chainansamit S, Chit-Uea-Ophat C, Reechaipichitkul W, Piromchai P. The diagnostic value of traditional nasal examination tools in an endoscopic era. Ear Nose Throat J. 2021;100(3):167-71.
3. Colavita L, Miraglia Del Giudice M, Stroscio G, Visalli C, Alterio T, Pidone C, et al. Allergic rhinitis and adenoid hypertrophy in children: is adenoidectomy always really useful? J Biol Regul Homeost Agents. 2015;29(2 Suppl 1):58-63.
4. da Lilly-Tariah OB, Aniemeka J. Plain radiological profile of paranasal sinuses in chronic nasal diseases in University of Port Harcourt Teaching Hospital. Niger J Med. 2006;15(3):305-8.
5. Klossek JM, Annesi-Maesano I, Pribil C, Didier A. The burden associated with ocular symptoms in allergic rhinitis. Int Arch Allergy Immunol. 2012;158(4):411-7.
6. K Maru Y, Gupta Y. Nasal Endoscopy Versus Other Diagnostic Tools in Sinonasal Diseases. Indian J Otolaryngol Head Neck Surg. 2016;68(2):202-6.
7. Neagos A, Dumitru M, Vrinceanu D, Costache A, Marinescu AN, Cergan R. Ultrasonography used in the diagnosis of chronic rhinosinusitis: From experimental imaging to clinical practice. Exp Ther Med. 2021;21(6):611.
8. Timmenga N, Stegenga B, Raghoebar G, van Hoogstraten J, van Weissenbruch R, Vissink A. The value of Waters' projection for assessing maxillary sinus inflammatory disease. Oral Surg Oral Med Oral Pathol Oral Radiol Endod. 2002; 93(1):103-9.

CHAPTER 7

Functional Assessment

Swikaar H Panchal

■ INTRODUCTION

Evaluation of a patient with allergic rhinitis begins with detailed history and examination. Apart from this, a thorough assessment of anatomy of the respiratory system which also includes ear, nose, and throat examination which is essential to rule out structural—congenital or acquired. At the same time, it is very important to objectively assess the functions of the respiratory system—both upper and lower airways. These tests correlate more with the quality of life of the patient, help us monitor the patient in our clinic in an objective manner as well as diagnose associated comorbidities such as asthma and obstructive sleep apnea (OSA). In this chapter, we have discussed regarding various tests to evaluate pulmonary functions. These tests can be further divided into tests for upper and lower airways.

- *Upper airway:* Peak nasal inspiratory flow (PNIF), rhinomanometry, rhinometry, and sleep studies
- *Lower airway:* Peak expiratory flow rate (PEFR), spirometry, and impulse oscillometry (IOS)

UPPER AIRWAY

Respiratory system starts at the nose and ends at the mitochondria where oxygen is utilized by the cell. Nose is the first part to expose to air from the atmosphere after which the air is filtered, humidified, and brought to body temperature before it reaches the oropharynx and lower airways. Nasal breathing conserves humidity as compared to oral breathing.

Nasal block is a predominant symptom in allergic rhinitis. It correlates with the quality of life of the patient. Symptoms told by patients as "cold" and "nasal stuffiness" could be vague and are better assessed objectively. Hence, it is important to evaluate air passage through the nasal cavity using objective parameters such as peak inspiratory flow, airflow resistance, and nasal patency. This can be achieved by using tests such as PNIF, rhinometry, and rhinomanometry. Each technique is unique and has its own set of advantages and disadvantages. They can be used alone or in combination. In reality, these are mainly used for research purposes. When used in clinical practice, they can give detailed idea about the functionality of the upper airway, especially the nose.

PEAK NASAL INSPIRATORY FLOW

Background

Peak nasal flows have been done from the time of peak expiratory flow (PEF) was done to monitor airway functions in asthma patients. Both inspiratory peak nasal inspiratory flow (PNIF) and peak nasal expiratory flow (PNEF) can be measured. Both of them correlate well are validated for assessment of nasal patency in adults. PNIF correlates better with obstructive nasal passage than PNEF. Some patients are uncomfortable with nasal secretions being blurted out and accumulating in the mask while performing expiratory maneuvers, and hence PNIF is more acceptable to patient than PNEF.

Peak nasal inspiratory flow is a portable, inexpensive, easy-to-use, and reliable technique to assess nasal patency in any patient. It has proven to be a reliable and a reproducible test which can be done easily. Normative data is available mainly for population >6 years of age all over the world. PNIF has been used as an objective tool in many diseases affecting the upper airway like allergic and nonallergic rhinitis, deviated nasal septum, nasal polyposis, adenotonsillar hypertrophy, etc.

Principle

Peak nasal flow helps evaluate nasal patency in an objective manner. It does not require any computer software for analysis. A patient is asked to exhale completely and start breathing from the residual volume, as hard and as fast from the nose, via a mask which is in connection to an inverted peak flow meter. The flow is recorded in liters per minute (L/min). It was observed in studies that patients demonstrated a "learning effect," i.e., their performance at doing PNIF improved with each attempt. Hence, by convention for measurement of PNIF, patients are asked to perform the test three times and the highest of the recordings taken as PNIF. Unilateral PNIF can also be done by occluding one of the nostrils. Although it has more applications in perioperative evaluations for instance in nasal septum deviation.

Device

- *Youlten's peak flow meter (Clement Clarke International Ltd., Mountain Ash, UK):* It looks similar to PEF meter, except for the part that it has a mask at the patient end. Flow meter should have a scale with minimum gradation of 10 L/min. Minimum value of PNIF recorded will be ≤30 L/min and maximum of ≥250 L/min **(Fig. 1)**.
- *Mask:* Cushioned anesthetic mask of appropriate size mask. The mask should form a tight seal around the nose and the mouth. It should be ensured that mask should not compress the cartilaginous part of the nose or cause any distortion to nasal cavity. The mask should not cause any

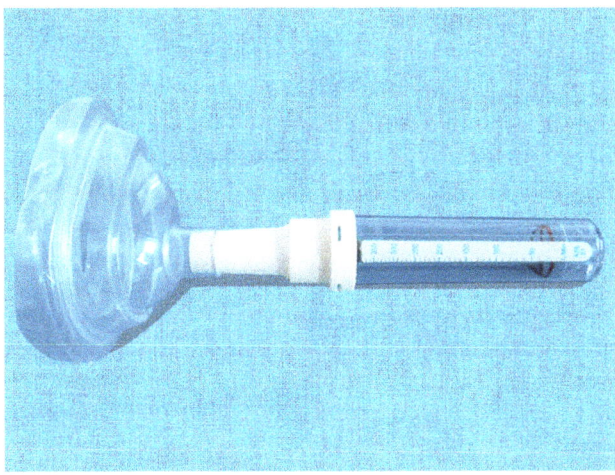

Fig. 1: Youlten's nasal peak flow meter.

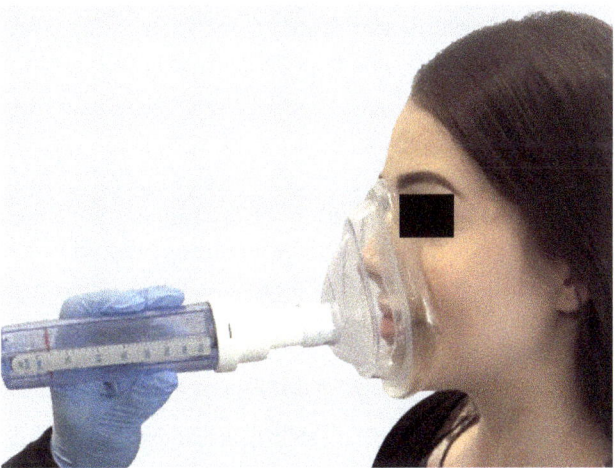

Fig. 2: Correct technique for placement of mask.

skin pulling or retraction. There should not be any leaks below or around the chin.

Technique

Patient is explained the procedure in details along with demonstration of correct technique. Consent is taken **(Fig. 2)**.

Prerequisites

- Detailed history and examination to be done.
- Gross structural abnormality of the nose and upper airways taken into consideration.

- It could be of value to perform a PEFR before performing the PNIF (as recommended by few authors).
- To ensure nasal cavity and the device are clean.
- No exercise 30 minutes prior to the test.
- Test to be performed in a standard setting with temperature 22°C.
- No oral decongestant (oral/topical) to be taken within 72 hours prior to test.
- Avoid performing test during exacerbations of illness, e.g., acute asthma.

Position: Test is performed in sitting position with back straight. It is recommended that only one method should be followed for all patients to have uniform results.

Maneuver: Residual Volume Technique

After being seated comfortably, patient is asked to exhale completely and take a deep breath with full force through the nose, keeping the mouth closed. This is called residual volume technique. Three such readings are taken and maximum of these reading is taken as PNIF. In case of error in method, an additional reading is recorded.

Validity of the Test

The readings are considered valid only if the discrepancy between the highest readings is not >10%, i.e., two of the highest readings should be within 10% of each other. To ensure recording of reliable data, it is prudent to perform the test under identical circumstances and in a standardized manner.

Interpretation

Cutoff for normal breathing: PNIF ≥ 140 L/min (likely to be normal)

Nasal obstruction is more likely when values are ≤90 L/min.

The above values can be used as rough guide for monitoring. It would be useful to refer to age-wise and region-wise charts to monitor for nasal patency. The readings of patients are compared with normative data and plotted as per centiles. Normative regional and age-wise date is available. Although there are no absolute values of normality and the patient is the best judge for evaluating changes.

A minimal value of 20 L/min is kept as a cutoff for significant clinical change post therapy.

Factors Affecting Peak Nasal Inspiratory Flow

- *Age:* It is shown in various studies that PNIF increases with age from childhood to adulthood and declines in older ages.

- *Height:* PNIF values correlate more with the height than age of the patient. PNIF increases with increasing height. In an Indian study, it was shown that if height increases by 1 unit, PNIF rises by 0.945 units.
- *Gender:* In adults, PNIF is higher in males than females. In children, correlation was found between gender and PNIF.
- *Race and ethnicity:* It was noted in various studies that racial differences also had an impact on PNIF values. It was attributed to variability in structure and modeling of the nose and upper airway.
- *Anatomical variations:* Structural alterations, such as deviated nasal septum, nasal spur, and polyp can alter PNIF values. PNIF may also vary due to anatomical abnormalities that can affect chest wall compliance. Normal structural variations contributed by racial differences have been described earlier. Unilateral obstructive pathologies can give false low PNIF values. In such scenarios, unilateral PNIF of the normal side may give a near accurate idea about nasal patency.
- *Lower airway functions:* There is a continuity between upper and lower airway. Hence, any abnormality of the lower airways will reflect in upper airways functions. For example, patients with emphysematous lungs may not be able to perform the nasal inspiratory maneuver effectively despite nasal patency being normal. This could give a false-low PNIF value.

Limitations
- Effort dependent
- Its measurement can be affected by severe dynamic nasal valve collapse
- It cannot be measured in severe obstructions.

Application of Peak Nasal Inspiratory Flow in Allergic Rhinitis
- Helps to correlate with quality of life of patient with AR.
- Objective assessment of nasal patency
- *Helps to identify disease phenotype:* Blockers from runners.
- Evaluation and monitoring the disease
- To evaluate response to therapy—intranasal corticosteroids, biologics, and immunotherapy
- Only test which can be done at home for monitoring of disease activity.

■ RHINOMETRY

Background
Acoustic rhinometry (AcR) is a commonly used technical method for examining nasal airway geometry with airflow dynamics and helps assess nasal patency in an objective manner. Measurements of AcR correlate well

with the subjective feeling of nasal obstruction as well as with imaging such as MRI and CT scan.

Principle

Acoustic rhinometry uses the "Bat Principle" in the nose. It is a passive method which works on the principle of acoustic reflections (echo), where sound impulse emission is used to determine the cross-sectional area (CSA) and volume of the nasal cavity. It is similar to the Doppler principle where sound waves emitted from a device are reflected back by structures which are picked up by the transducers. The reflected frequencies undergo processing and conversion to electrical signals which can be interpreted. In AcR, an acoustic wave is generated by a sound generator through a tubular device attached to one of the nasal openings. The reflected waves are picked by a transducer on the same device and compared with the incident wave. As quoted by Hilberg in his work on acoustic rhinometry—if the size of the entrance to airways is known, the size of the reflections may reflect changes of the airway size. The time between the reflections may give the distance between the changes dependent on the speed of sound. Hence, it would be possible to determine the area as a function of distance in the airways. It can give numerical information such as the CSA at certain distances and volumes between certain points in the nose. This gives a good idea about the geometry of the nose, but may not give the exact cause of narrowing **(Fig. 3)**.

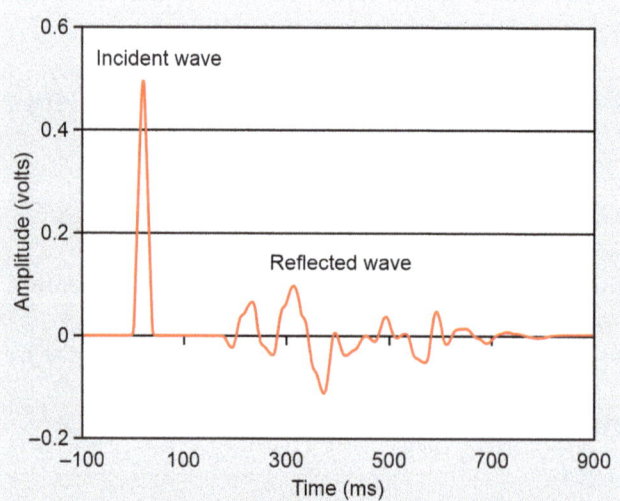

Fig. 3: The reflected signal from nasal cavity.
Source: Hilberg O. Objective measurement of nasal airway dimensions using acoustic rhinometry: methodological and clinical aspects. Allergy. 2002;57 Suppl 70:5-39.

In a tube system with one-dimensional sound propagation, changes in the acoustic impedance are directly proportionate to changes in the CSA. Due to advancement in computers and technology, it is now possible to sample, store, and calculate the reflections. **Figure 3** depicts the reflection pattern of an incident pulse from a tube with multiple changes in acoustic impedance CSA.

The reflected wave collected by the receiver is still data in the form of frequencies. Hence, a Fourier and inverse Fourier analysis needs to be done for further analysis of the data.

Equipment Needed for Acoustic Rhinomanometry (Figs. 4A to D)

- Microphone (sound generator) located in the sonic tube
- Nasal adapters

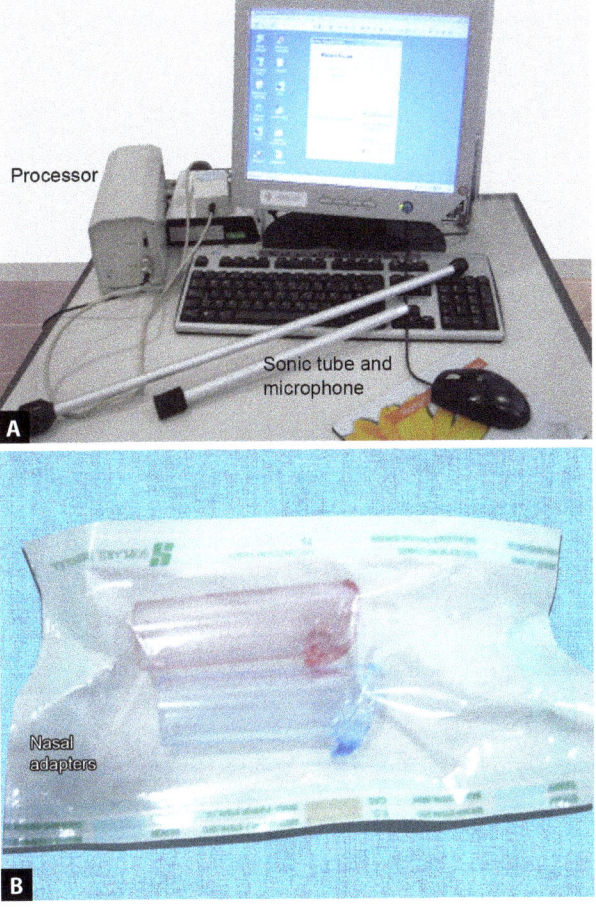

Figs. 4A and B

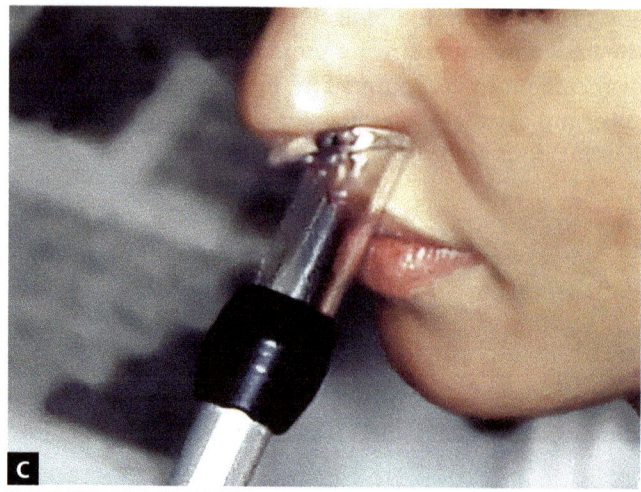

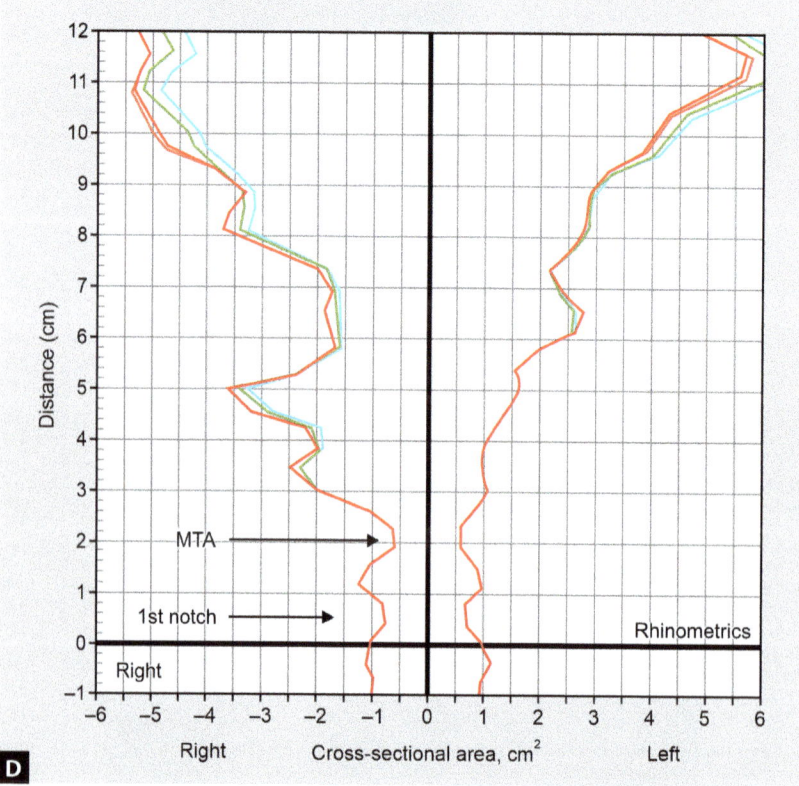

Figs. 4C and D

Figs. 4A to D: Equipment for acoustic rhinometry (AcR): (A) Basic hardware, microphone in the sonic tube; (B) Nasal adapters; (C) An intermediate piece or adapter that is applied to nasal window, which is then connected to sonic tube; and (D) AcR graph. (MTA: minimum transverse area)

- An intermediate piece or adapter is applied in the nasal window, which in turn is connected to the sonic tube. The adapter has a constant and preset length and section.
- Computer
- Technical expert to conduct the test

Acoustic Rhinometry Curve

The clinical implication of AcR is in the ability to measure CSA of the nasal passage to evaluate nasal patency. Acoustic rhinomanometry converts sound impulses reflected by nasal cavity into waves which represent CSA as function of distance. This curve provides with data regarding degree of nasal obstruction **(Fig. 5)**.

Area distance curve usually shows minimum of three notches, each representing narrowest portion of the nasal cavity.

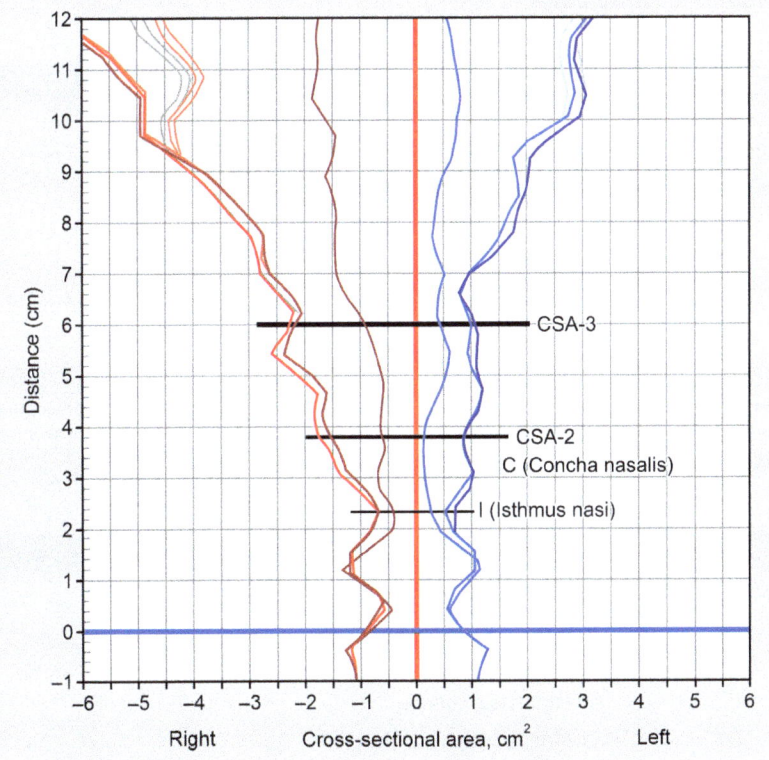

Fig. 5: Example of acoustic rhinometry (AcR) curve.
Source: Krzych-Fałta E, Kaczyńska O, Samoliński B, Sybilski A. A new perspective on acoustic rhinometry in terms of standardisation, including the nasal allergen provocation test. Postepy Dermatol Alergol. 2022;39(5):852-5.

Interpretation of the Acoustic Rhinometry Curve

Before interpretation it is important to understand the components of the AR curve. It is a graphical representation in two-dimensions.

X-axis represents the extent of the nasal cavity evaluated. It is measured from the anterior most part of nasal opening till the nasopharynx. It is measured in centimeters.

The Y-axis represents the CSA of the nasal cavity at each point along the X-axis, usually measured in square centimeters. This axis depicts the diameter of the nasal passage at various points.

The curve is plotted automatically using the computer algorithm. It represents the change in the CSA across the nasal passage. Points have been described in the **Tables 1 and 2**.

Procedure

- Patient is explained about the details of the procedure and written informed consent taken.

TABLE 1: Different points on the AR curve.

Point on AR curve	Anatomical correlate	Significance
0 (zero)	The start of the nasal cavity	-
I	The nasal isthmus (isthmus nasi)	First narrowing of nasal cavity
C	The head of the inferior nasal concha (concha nasalis)	Second narrowing of nasal cavity
E	Distal section of head if inferior basal concha	-

Source: Krzych-Fałta E, Kaczyńska O, Samoliński B, Sybilski A. A new perspective on acoustic rhinometry in terms of standardisation, including the nasal allergen provocation test. Postepy Dermatol Alergol. 2022;39(5):852-5.

TABLE 2: Areas at the above points.

Areas	Anatomical correlate
0-I	Vestibule of the nose
I-C	The distance between the nasal isthmus and the head of the inferior nasal concha
C-E	The end of the nasal concha
E-G	Nasopharynx space

Source: Krzych-Fałta E, Kaczyńska O, Samoliński B, Sybilski A. A new perspective on acoustic rhinometry in terms of standardisation, including the nasal allergen provocation test. Postepy Dermatol Alergol. 2022;39(5):852-5.

- Test is to be done is a quiet room (free of ambient noise, <60 dB to 50 dB).
- Prior to test patient needs to clear his nose of all secretions as much as possible
- To ensure that patient is well rested and calm. No exercise has been performed at least 15-20 minutes prior to performing test.
- To ensure no local or systemic drugs are taken which can affect nasal mucosa.
- Test is done in sitting upright position.
- Patient is asked to keep his/her head in upright position. Using a head frame to keep the head in a more rigid fixed position has not helped much and has affected the repeatability. Hence not recommended.
- The nasal adapter (appropriate size) connected to the rhinometry probe is place at the opening of one of the nostrils. Sometimes, water-soluble gel or soft paraffin wax may be applied around the probe to ensure airtight seal.
- It is important to ensure that the angle of the acoustic rhinomanometry probe is proper in line with the nasal cavity as it affects the quality of results. Technical expertise is required for same.
- The measurements are made mainly during breath-holding, as breathing may interfere with acoustic signals. The test is passive and does not require the patient to perform any complex maneuvers.
- During each session, three consecutive measurements are conducted for each nasal passage, and their average is calculated. This process is typically accompanied by the application of an intranasal decongestant, followed by additional measurements after the decongestant has taken effect.
- *Congestion factor* is calculated as a percent change in the predecongestant and postdecongestant area and volume measurements. It is given by a formula:

$$\text{Congestion factor} = \frac{(\text{Postdecongested area or volume}) - (\text{Predecongested area or volume})}{(\text{Predecongested area or volume})}$$

Using the above factor, the nasal obstruction can be graded relatively as normal, mild, moderate, severe, and markedly severe.

Factors Affecting Acoustic Rhinometry

- *Nasal air leaks:* Nasal air leaks can cause erroneous results and poor repeatability of the test. Most common cause is the nasal probe not fitting snuggly in the nasal opening. Water-soluble gel or soft paraffin wax can be used to prevent this.

- *Diurnal variations and nasal cycle:* It is a well-known fact that airflow through each nostril is very closely regulated by the various physiological factors which control the nasal cycle. The nasal cycle influences the airflow via alternate congestion and decongestion of nasal mucosa of each side. Autonomic nervous system is a major regulator of nasal cycle, so is the hypothalamus. Hence, even diurnal variations affect the readings of AcR. Hence, it is important that test should be repeated at the same time of the day as the previous reading.

    Because a classic nasal cycle is associated with alternating congestion/decongestion cycles matched by the opposite in the other nostril, the sum of the two sides is usually constant.
- *Ethnicity, regional, and racial differences:* Variability was noted in AcR curves of various races considering the fact that different races have different geometrical structure of nose.
- *External dimensions of nose:* Minimum cross-sectional area (MCA) has correlation with external nasal dimensions.
- *Age, weight, height, and body weight:* Weak correlation was found with MCA.
- *Structural alterations in nasal mucosa:* Any change in internal anatomy and mucosal alterations can affect AcR curve. Deviated septum, polyp, and spur can distort normal AcR curve. One way to differentiate mucosal alteration from structural ones is by administration of nasal decongestant. Postdecongestant and mucosal anomalies such as edema will normalize or change whereas, anatomical defects will not.
- *Exercise:* Nasal mucosal structure is affected by exercise. Exercise causes increased sympathetic drive leading to nasal decongestion. Hence, it is important that the patient is well rested at least 15–20 minutes after exercise, before proceeding with AcR.
- *Distance from the nasal inlet:* It is indicated by studies that measurements as far as 6 cm from the nasal entrance are accurate. There is acoustic distortion in the more posterior aspects of nose due to the sound getting lost along the maxillary sinus ostia and the osteomeatal complex. Hence, the measurements are more accurate in anterior 0–5 cm of nasal cavity **(Fig. 6)**.

Applications in Allergic Rhinitis

- *Evaluation and examination of nasal anatomy in patients with allergic rhinitis:* Measures volume and minimum cross sectional area-MCA in patients with allergic rhinitis.
- *Evaluation of therapeutic interventions:* AcR helps in evaluating effect of various treatment modalities in patients with allergic rhinitis. This

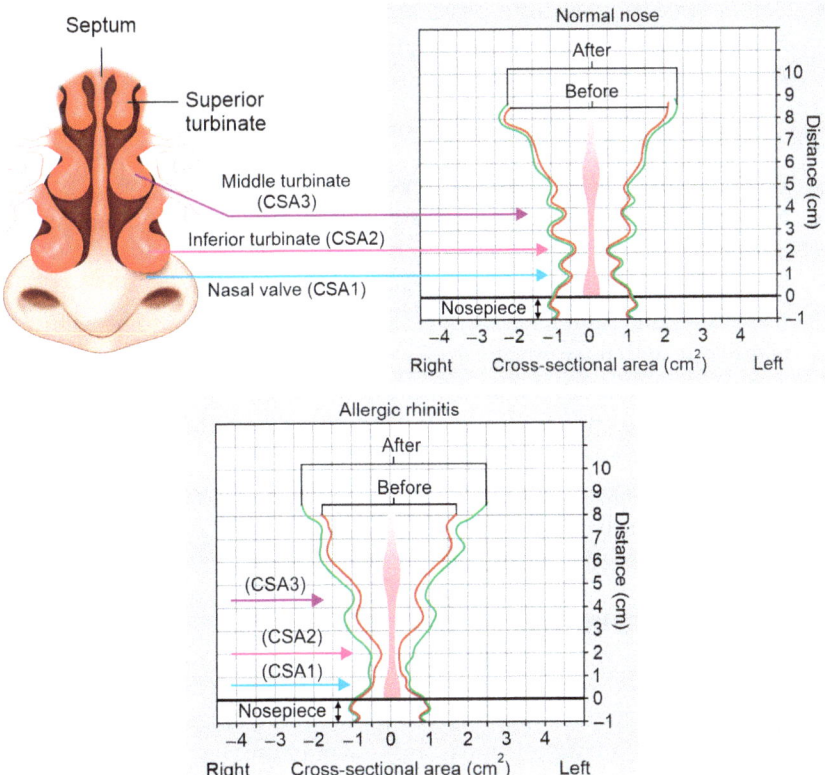

Fig. 6: Normal anatomy of the nose with corresponding acoustic rhinometry (AcR) curve showing pre- and postdecongestant effect. Image lower shows AcR curve in patient with allergic rhinitis. Note the postcongestion readings show hardly any variability at points cross-sectional area (CSA)-1, 2, or 3 signifying anatomical landmarks.
Source: Uzzaman A, Metcalfe DD, Komarow HD. Acoustic rhinometry in the practice of allergy. Ann Allergy Asthma Immunol. 2006;97(6):745-51; quiz 751-2, 799.

includes effect of pre- and postnasal decongestants and intranasal corticosteroids. It also helps quantify the response to therapy.
- It has a role in nasal provocation testing.
- It helps in objectifying symptoms of nasal blockage and hence identifies blockers.
- *Occupational exposures:* It helps to evaluate the effect of dust, chemical compounds, smoke at work place, and helps point toward a triggering factor toward rhinitis or asthma.
- *Sleep disordered breathing:* Techniques of AcR can be applied to evaluate comorbidities such as OSA and snoring where nasal dimensions can give a clue regarding site of fixed or variable obstruction.

- *AcR in infants:* It has been possible now to perform AcR in infants using miniprobes. The Miniprobe has a flexible shaft, the end of which has a circular tip that forms a tight seal with the infant's nose.

Limitations
- Procuring the AcR equipment can be a costly affair.
- Needs to have technical expertise and training to run and maintain the device.
- Needs very good patient cooperation and compliance. Patients with respiratory difficulties, nasal congestion, or discomfort may have difficulty complying with the procedure, affecting the reliability of the results.
- AcR gives idea about the area and volume of the nasal cavity; although it does not give any idea about the underlying nasal mucosal pathology. Hence, it cannot point toward an etiology.
- AcR is a passive test. Hence, it cannot give dynamic assessment of airflow through the nasal cavity.
- It cannot give a fair assessment of nasal valve area.

■ RHINOMANOMETRY

Background
The various parameters to study nasal patency were nasal volume and pressure. The early attempts to measure nasal pressure were made by Donders in 1859. He sealed off one of the nostrils with a mercury manometer while active respiration. Since those times nasal or rhinomanometry has come a long way. Rhinomanometry is the study to quantify nasal airway resistance. It is a well-accepted method all over.

Principle
Rhinomanometry measures the pressure encountered by air passing through the nasal cavity. It uses specialized equipment to measure airflow and resistance while the patient is breathing.

For understanding basic principles of rhinomanometry, it is vital to understand the nasal cycle. The objective assessment of nasal patency as well as its correlation to subjective feeling of nasal patency or nose block is not solely dependent on resistance of the nasal passages. The occurrence of turbulent flows also plays a role.

Rhinomanometry may be of various types depending on:
- The position of the probe—anterior or posterior
- Depending on patient effort—active or passive

Anterior rhinomanometry: When the measurement systems are places anteriorly to nose or at level of nasal openings.

Posterior rhinomanometry: It requires placement of an intraoral device to detect choanal pressure.

Note: Both of the above methods can be active or passive depending on whether patient is breathing spontaneously (active) or whether patient is asked to hold breath and a predetermined flow is made to pass through the nasal passage using a special device (passive).

Anterior rhinomanometry: It is used to measure unilateral and total nasal conductance. Conductance is the airflow through the nose at a sample pressure of 75 Pa. Conductance is a better measure than resistance as in case of complete blockage, resistance tends toward infinity whereas conductance will tend toward zero and would be easy to calibrate and measure.

Nasal resistance is predetermined at a fixed pressure of 150 Kpa.

Four-phase Rhinomanometry

Here the conductance is calculated in four phases of breathing. Although the results are not different from normal rhinometry.

Equipment Required

- *Rhinometry machine:* This device measures nasal airflow and pressure. It consists of a pressure transducer, airflow sensor, and computer interface. Standardized equipment as per consensus guidelines is available.
- *Mask:* Recently, masks have also been recommended where the noninvestigated side is blocked by a tape without distortion of nasal inlet.

Procedure

- The patient is explained about the procedure.
- Test is performed in sitting position.
- Patients asked to clear their nose before each session of measuring resistance.
- All equipment is calibrated before each test run for a patient.
- A face mask is applied to the patient which forms a seal around the nose, with the patient breathing through a flow head attached to it. Inside the mouth, a pressure-sensing tube detects pressure in the posterior nares when airflow is directed toward the mouth. Total nasal airflow can be measured from both nostrils, or separately from each nostril by blocking one side.
- In active anterior rhinomanometry, the pressure-sensing tube is typically taped to one nasal passage, allowing separate measurements **(Fig. 7)**.

Rhinomanometry has similar applications as rhinometry in patients with allergic rhinitis.

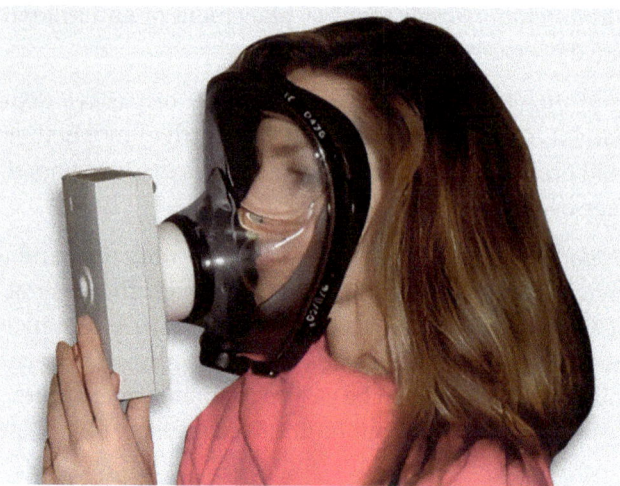

Fig. 7: Performing anterior rhinomanometry.
Source: Ottaviano G, Fokkens WJ. Measurements of nasal airflow and patency: a critical review with emphasis on the use of peak nasal inspiratory flow in daily practice. Allergy. 2016;71:162-74.

Confounding Factors Affecting Usage of Rhinomanometry

- *Complex and high maintenance equipment:* It is used mainly only for research purposes.
- Presence of mucous in nasal passage can lead to false results of obstruction.
- Nasal cycle is dynamic and constantly changing, hence values of nasal resistance can be unstable and unreliable **(Figs. 8A to D)**.

Table 3 summarizes and compares various methods to assess nasal patency.

■ SLEEP STUDIES IN ALLERGIC RHINITIS

Sleep studies, particularly polysomnography (PSG), can play a significant role in assessing the impact on quality of sleep of patients with allergic rhinitis. It also helps in identifying potential sleep-related disorders that may coexist with allergic rhinitis. In this section, we will only discuss regarding the role of polysomnography in patients with allergic rhinitis.

- *Identification of sleep disturbances:* Patients with AR commonly present with nasal congestion, which can disrupt normal breathing patterns during sleep, leading to sleep disturbances. Sleep studies can help identify these disturbances, such as snoring, mouth breathing, and OSA.
- *Assessment of sleep quality:* Sleep studies provide objective measures of sleep architecture, including total sleep time, sleep efficiency, and sleep stages. Patients with allergic rhinitis may experience fragmented sleep

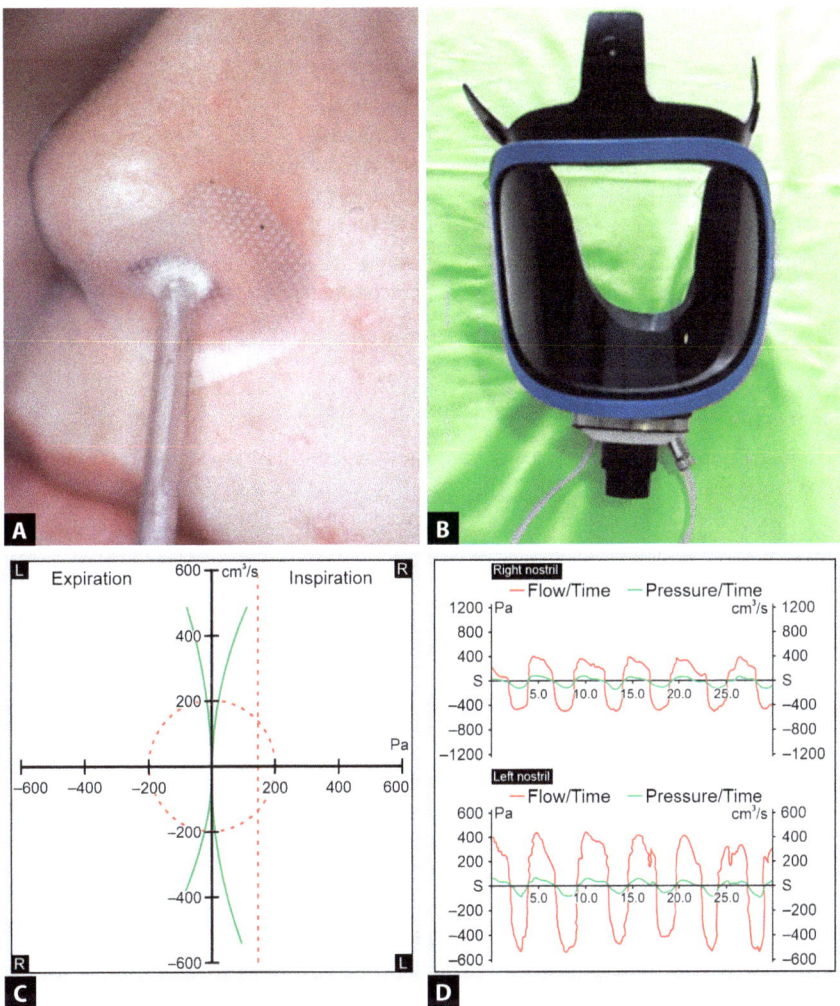

Figs. 8A to D: Active anterior rhinomanometry: (A) Adhesive tape with nasal cannula measuring pressure; (B) Face mask; (C) XY recording axis; and (D) Sinusoidal oscillography.
Source: Valero A, Navarro AM, Del Cuvillo A, Alobid I, Benito JR, Colás C, et al. Position paper on nasal obstruction: evaluation and treatment. J Investig Allergol Clin Immunol. 2018;28(2):67-90.

due to nasal congestion, leading to decreased sleep quality. Sleep studies can quantify these disruptions and their impact on overall sleep quality.
- *Evaluation of nasal airway resistance:* Nasal congestion is a hallmark symptom of allergic rhinitis which can increase nasal airway resistance during sleep, leading to breathing difficulties. Sleep studies can assess nasal airway resistance and airflow dynamics during sleep, providing

TABLE 3: Comparison between various modalities for assessment of nasal patency.

Characteristics	PNIF	Rhinomanometry	Acoustic rhinometry
Definition	Device with a scale to measure nasal airflow and a nasal mask	Transducers that measure nasal airflow and differences in nasal pressure	Principle of ultrasound
Measurement	Nasal flows in liters per minute during maximal inspiration	Nasal resistance and conductance	Cross section and volume between two points of the nasal cavity
Patient cooperation	Yes	Yes	Minimum
Useful for nasal challenge test	Yes	Yes	Yes
Useful for medical treatment evaluation	Yes	Yes	Yes
Useful for surgical treatment evaluation	Yes	Yes	Yes
Strengths	Portable; useful for home monitoring of patient's treatment	Still the "golden standard" for measurement of nasal obstruction	Most used in children; guidelines for its use in nasal challenge test
Drawbacks	Alar collapse; not useful when nose totally blocked	Relative high cost of equipment	Relative high cost of equipment

(PINF: peak nasal inspiratory flow)
Source: Ottaviano G, Fokkens WJ. Measurements of nasal airflow and patency: a critical review with emphasis on the use of peak nasal inspiratory flow in daily practice. Allergy. 2016;71:162-74.

insights into the severity of nasal obstruction and its impact on breathing patterns.
- *Detection of sleep-disordered breathing:* Allergic rhinitis is associated with an increased risk of sleep-disordered breathing such as OSA. Sleep studies can detect the presence of OSA by monitoring respiratory parameters, including apnea-hypopnea index (AHI), oxygen saturation levels, and respiratory effort. Identifying OSA in patients with allergic rhinitis is crucial as it may require specific management strategies, including continuous positive airway pressure (CPAP) therapy.

- *Assessment of treatment response:* Sleep studies can evaluate the effectiveness of treatment interventions for allergic rhinitis, such as intranasal corticosteroids or antihistamines, in improving sleep quality and reducing sleep disturbances. Objective measures obtained from sleep studies, such as AHI and sleep efficiency, can assess treatment response over time.

Overall, sleep studies play a valuable role in assessing the impact of allergic rhinitis on sleep quality, identifying sleep-related disorders, and guiding treatment decisions to optimize patient care.

LOWER AIRWAY

As per the "united airway" concept, nose and lungs are considered to be a continuum of the same anatomical and functional unit. It is because they share morphological, immunological, and pathological factors. Hence, in a patient with allergic rhinitis, it becomes all the most important to have a detailed evaluation of the lower airways as it is the part of the same functional unit. Nearly 40% of patients suffering from allergic rhinitis have asthma and around 80% of asthma patients have allergic rhinitis.

■ PEAK EXPIRATORY FLOW RATE

Background

Peak flow meter is simple, cost-effective, and a patient-friendly device which helps to evaluate PEFR in a patient with lower airway obstruction. PEFR is the maximum flow rate generated during a forceful exhalation, starting from the level for full inspiration or inspiratory reserve volume. The device is calibrated to measure flows in L/min.

Peak expiratory flow rate reflects flow through the proximal airways. It does not give much idea about the smaller airways **(Fig. 9)**.

Method to Perform Peak Expiratory Flow Rate

- *Prerequisites:*
  - Patient should be stable clinically, i.e., free from any breathing difficulty or not in a flare up.
  - Children >5 years are competent enough to be trained and to perform the maneuver.
- The PEFR maneuver is majorly effort dependent. Hence, it is of utmost importance that the patient understands the procedure well. Consent is taken.
- *Position:* Any position, standing or sitting with an erect back is preferred. It is important that subsequent readings should be taken in the same position by patient.

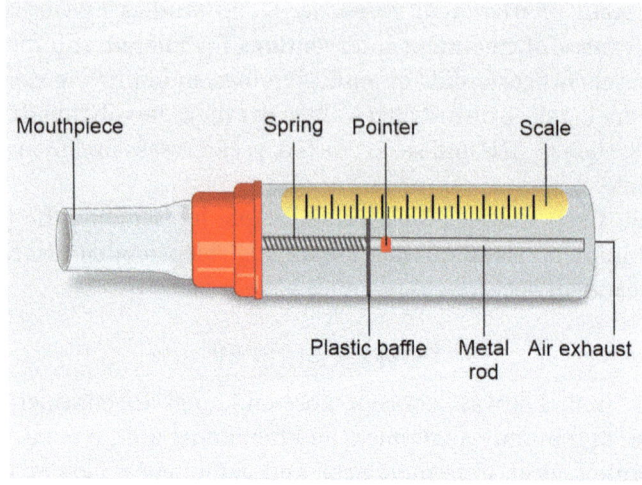

Fig. 9: Parts of peak flow meter.
Source: Booker R. Peak expiratory flow measurement. Nurs Stand. 2007;21(39):42-3.

- An appropriate size mouthpiece is taken. Such that it can be easily held in the mouth by the patient between the upper and lower incisors and encircled by lips to form a tight seal. There should be no leaks. Disposable mouthpieces can be used in office setup. Small pediatric size mouthpieces are also available.
- The pointer or marker is dragged down to the least value which is zero.
- Holding the device parallel to the ground, patient is asked to take a deep breath in and hold. The device is placed with the mouthpiece in the mouth in a manner that there is a tight seal and there are no leaks.
- Patient is then asked to breathe out forcefully through the mouth as hard and as fast as possible.
- Note is made of the reading from the peak flow meter.
- Same process is repeated twice and the highest of the three readings is taken as peak flow. It is to be ensured that while performing three readings that fatigue should not set in while recording as it can lead to false low readings.
- The readings are then compared with available nomograms which are age and height-wise for a particular population.

Calculation of diurnal variation in PEFR: The allergic process varies with the circadian rhythm of the body. It is mainly due to variations in plasma levels of histamines, steroids, and catecholamines with the sleep-wake cycle. Hence, PEFR values also differ with diurnal variations. The lowest PEFR for a patient is noted at around 4 AM in the morning.

Increased diurnal variation points toward increased disease activity or poor disease control.

It is calculated as follows:
- Twice daily readings are taken.
- PEFR variability calculated as:

$$\frac{(\text{Highest reading in daytime} - \text{Lowest reading}) \times 100}{\text{Mean of both values}}$$

Note: PEF variability >13% is considered significant.
- *Assessment of respiratory function:* PEF meters help evaluate the maximum airflow during forced expiration, aiding in assessing respiratory function in individuals with allergic rhinitis, especially those with coexisting asthma.
- *Monitoring asthma symptoms:* PEF measurements track changes in lung function and asthma symptoms over time, particularly in allergic rhinitis patients with asthma. Fluctuations in PEF readings can indicate worsening asthma control or exacerbations triggered by allergic rhinitis symptoms.
- *Assessment of treatment response:* PEF meters evaluate the response to asthma and allergic rhinitis treatments, including bronchodilators, corticosteroids, and allergy medications. Improvements in PEF values indicate effective management of both conditions.
- *Patient home and self-management:* Teaching allergic rhinitis patients how to use PEF meters empowers them to actively participate in managing their respiratory health. Regular PEF monitoring enables individuals to recognize early signs exacerbations or allergic reactions and take appropriate action.
- *Before performing PNIF:* It is done to rule out lower airways obstruction which can give false low reading of PNIF.

■ SPIROMETRY

Background

Spirometry plays a crucial role in the comprehensive evaluation and management of patients with allergic rhinitis. Spirometry is the measurement of lung volumes during forced expiratory and tidal maneuvers done by the patient.

Role of Spirometry in Allergic Rhinitis

The "One Airway, One Disease" concept establishes that a patient with allergic rhinitis along with upper airway can have at least some disease process affecting the lower airways too. Although the amount of predisposition varies, a patient with allergic rhinitis has a concomitant underlying asthma or progresses to develop asthma in later life. Hence, it becomes important in patients with allergic rhinitis to have a spirometry done. General practitioners and ENT are first contact or only treating doctors to majority of patients with allergic rhinitis. In such a scenario asthma may go underdiagnosed. Stressing on this particular aspect, any patient with allergic rhinitis must undergo spirometry to evaluate lower airway functions and pick up underlying asthma. Also, spirometry should be done in all patients with symptoms such as cough or other symptoms pointing toward lower airway involvement. In few studies, it has been demonstrated that patients who were treated for both upper and lower airway involvement (on diagnosis), had better quality of life than ones treated for only allergic rhinitis. Hence, spirometry can help diagnose and monitor asthma in patients with allergic rhinitis and pave the way for better management of patients **(Fig. 10)**.

- *Measurement of baseline respiratory parameters diagnose asthmatics:* Spirometry provides baseline measurements of lung function, including forced expiratory volume in one second (FEV1) and forced vital capacity (FVC), allowing for the evaluation of respiratory health in allergic rhinitis patients.
- Assessment of treatment response in patients with asthma and allergic rhinitis

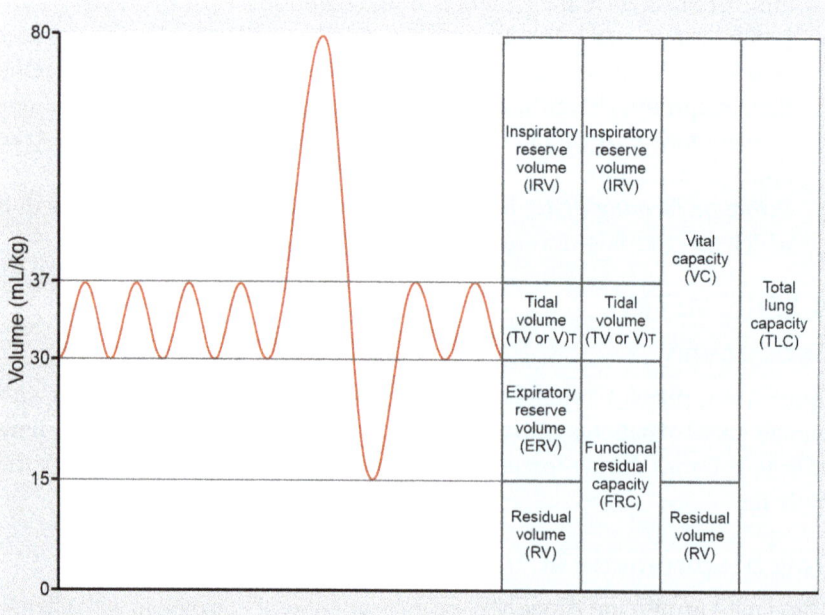

Fig. 10: Spirometry: basic lung volumes and capacities.
Source: Erratum: "Spirometry: step by step". V.C. Moore. Breathe 2012;8:232-40. Breathe (Sheff). 2022;18(3):115217.

- Evaluation of treatment response to inhaled corticosteroids, biologics, and immunotherapy from time to time.
- Optimization of treatment regimen
- Monitoring of disease activity

■ KEY POINTS

- Tests for upper airways include various tests to evaluate nasal patency and airway resistance across the nose—PNIF, rhinometry, rhinomanometry, and sleep studies.
- PNIF is a very simple, inexpensive, reliable, and reproducible test which can be used to evaluate nasal patency, monitor disease activity, and response to treatment at home as well as outpatient department.
- AcR uses the principle of acoustic reflections to assess the CSA and volume of the nasal cavity. Although it has wide applications in patients with allergic rhinitis, AcR equipment is expensive and requires technical expertise.
- Rhinomanometry is another modality which measures the pressure across the nasal airway passage to understand airway dynamics and resistance in allergic rhinitis. This technique uses a complicated algorithm, not very user-friendly, hence mainly has role in research.
- Although allergic rhinitis is a disease involving nose, owing to the "United Airway" concept and to rule out comorbidities such as asthma and OSA, it is important to perform tests for lower airways too. They include PEFR and spirometry.

■ SUGGESTED READING

1. Baraniuk JN, Ali M, Naranch K. Hypertonic saline nasal provocation and acoustic rhinometry. Clin Exp Allergy. 2002;32:543-50.
2. Booker R. Peak expiratory flow measurement. Nurs Stand. 2007;21(39):42-3.
3. Clement PA, Hirsch C. Rhinomanometry—a review. ORL J Otorhinolaryngol Relat Spec. 1984;46(4):173-91.
4. Clement PAR, Gordts F, Standardisation Committee on Objective Assessment of the Nasal Airway, IRS, and ERS. Consensus report on acoustic rhinometry and rhinomanometry. Rhinology. 2005;43:169-79.
5. Corey JP, Gungor A, Nelson R, Liu X, Fredberg J. Normative standards for nasal cross-sectional areas by race as measured by acoustic rhinometry. Otolaryngol Head Neck Surg. 1998;119:389-93.
6. Dahl R, Nielsen LP, Kips J, Foresi A, Howarth P, Richards DH, et al. Intranasal and inhaled fluticasone propionate for pollen-induced rhinitis and asthma. Allergy. 2006;60:875-81.
7. Das M, Sabui TK, Ahuja N. (2021). Reference Value of Nasal Peak Inspiratory Flow Rate in Indian Children: A Cross-sectional Study. J Clin Diagn Res. 2021;15(7):SC05-SC0710.

8. Djupesland PG, Lyholm B. Nasal airway dimensions in term neonates measured by continuous wide-band noise acoustic rhinometry. Acta Otolaryngol. 1997;117:424-32.
9. Djupesland PG, Lyholm B. Technical abilities and limitations of acoustic rhinometry optimised for infants. Rhinology. 1998;36(3):104-13.
10. Enberg RN, Ownby DR. Peak nasal inspiratory flow and Wright peak flow: a comparison of their reproducibility. Ann Allergy. 1991;67:371-4.
11. Erratum: "Spirometry: step by step". V.C. Moore. Breathe 2012;8:232-40. Breathe (Sheff). 2022;18(3):115217.
12. Faber CE, Grymer L. Available techniques for objective assessment of upper airway narrowing in snoring and sleep apnea. Sleep Breath. 2003;7:77-86.
13. Gilain L, Coste A, Ricolfi F, Dahan E, Marliac D, Peynegre R, et al. Nasal cavity geometry measured by acoustic rhinometry and computed tomography. Arch Otolaryngol Head Neck Surg. 1997;123:401-5.
14. Gurr P, Diver J, Morgan N, MacGregor F, Lund V. Acoustic rhinometry of the Indian and Anglo-Saxon nose. Rhinology. 1996;34:156-9.
15. Hamilton JW, Cook JA, Phillips DE, Jones AS. Limitations of acoustic rhinometry determined by a simple model. Acta Otolaryngol. 1995;115(6):811-4.
16. Hilberg O, Grymer LF, Pedersen OF. Spontaneous variations in congestion of the nasal mucosa. Ann Allergy Asthma Immunol. 1995;74:516-21.
17. Hilberg O, Jackson AC, Swift DL, Pedersen OF. Acoustic rhinometry: evaluation of nasal cavity geometry by acoustic reflection. J Appl Physiol (1985). 1989;66(1):295-303.
18. Hilberg O, Jensen FT, Pedersen OF. Nasal airway geometry: comparison between acoustic reflections and magnetic resonance scanning. J Appl Physiol. 1993;75:2811-9.
19. Hilberg O, Pedersen OF. Acoustic rhinometry: influence of paranasal sinuses. J Appl Physiol. 1996;80:1589-94.
20. Hilberg O, Pedersen OF. Acoustic rhinometry: recommendations for technical specifications and standard operating procedures. Rhinol Suppl. 2000;16:3-17.
21. Hilberg O. Objective measurement of nasal airway dimensions using acoustic rhinometry: methodological and clinical aspects. Allergy. 2002;57 Suppl 70:5-39.
22. Holmstrom M, Scadding GK, Lund VJ, Darby YC. Assessment of nasal obstruction. A comparison between rhinomanometry and nasal inspiratory peak flow. Rhinology. 1990;28:191-6.
23. Jones AS, Viani L, Phillips D, Charters P. The objective assessment of nasal patency. Clin Otolaryngol Allied Sci. 1991;16:206-11.
24. Krzych-Fałta E, Kaczyńska O, Samoliński B, Sybilski A. A new perspective on acoustic rhinometry in terms of standardisation, including the nasal allergen provocation test. Postepy Dermatol Alergol. 2022;39(5):852-5.
25. Lenders H, Scholl R, Brunner M. Acoustic rhinometry: the bat principle of the nose [in German]. HNO 1992;40:239-47
26. Maeda Y, Okita W, Ichimura K. Increased nasal patency caused by smoking and contraction of isolated human nasal mucosa. Rhinology. 2004;42:63-7.
27. Mamikoglu B, Houser SM, Corey JP. An interpretation method for objective assessment of nasal congestion with acoustic rhinometry. Laryngoscope. 2002;112:926-9.

28. Morgan NJ, MacGregor FB, Birchall MA, Lund VJ, Sittampalam Y. Racial differences in nasal fossa dimensions determined by acoustic rhinometry. Rhinology. 1995;33:224-8.
29. Morris LG, Burschtin O, Lebowitz RA, Jacobs JB, Lee KC. Nasal obstruction and sleep-disordered breathing: a study using acoustic rhinometry. Am J Rhinol. 2005;19:33-9.
30. Mo S, Gupta SS, Stroud A, Strazdins E, Hamizan AW, Rimmer J, et al. Nasal peak inspiratory flow in healthy and obstructed patients: systematic review and meta-analysis. Laryngoscope. 2021;131(2):260-7.
31. Nagaraju MK. 32 Peak Nasal Inspiratory Flow Levels in Children With Allergic Rhinitis and Their Health Related Quality of Life (HRQL). World Allergy Organ J. 2012;5(Suppl 2):S28.
32. Nathan RA, Eccles R, Howarth PH, Steinsvåg SK, Togias A. Objective monitoring of nasal patency and nasal physiology in rhinitis. J Allergy Clin Immunol. 2005;115(3 Suppl. 1):S442-59.
33. Ottaviano G, Fokkens WJ. Measurements of nasal airflow and patency: a critical review with emphasis on the use of peak nasal inspiratory flow in daily practice. Allergy. 2016;71:162-74.
34. Phagoo SB, Watson RA, Pride NB. Use of nasal peak flow to assess nasal patency. Allergy. 1997;52:901-8.
35. Sikorska-Szaflik H, Sozańska B. Peak nasal inspiratory flow in children with allergic rhinitis. Is it related to the quality of life? Allergol Immunopathol (Madr). 2020;48(2):187-93.
36. Sipila J, Nyberg-Simola S, Suonpaa J, Laippala P. Some fundamental studies on clinical measurement conditions in acoustic rhinometry. Rhinology. 1996;34:206-9.
37. Sonawane NS, Gour SM, Munje RP, Vandana PB. Spirometric evaluation in patients with allergic rhinitis-emphasising need of early diagnosis: a tertiary care experience from Central India. Int J Adv Med. 2018;5:1460-4.
38. Taylor G, Macneil AR, Freed DL. Assessing degree of nasal patency by measuring peak expiratory flow rate through the nose. J Allergy Clin Immunol. 1973;52:193-8.
39. Teixeira RUF, Zappelini CEM, Alves FS, da Costa EA. Peak nasal inspiratory flow evaluation as an objective method of measuring nasal airflow. Braz J Otorhinolaryngol 2011;77:473-80.
40. Uzzaman A, Metcalfe DD, Komarow HD. Acoustic rhinometry in the practice of allergy. Ann Allergy Asthma Immunol. 2006;97(6):745-51; quiz 751-2, 799.
41. Valero A, Navarro AM, Del Cuvillo A, Alobid I, Benito JR, Colás C, et al. Position paper on nasal obstruction: evaluation and treatment. J Investig Allergol Clin Immunol. 2018;28(2):67-90.
42. Waheeda S, Syed Liyakath AS, Sathyamurthy K. Evaluation of Pulmonary Function Tests in Allergic Rhinitis Patients Attending a Rural Tertiary Care Hospital in South India. J Sci Soc. 2022;49(1):25-7.
43. Wilson AM, Fowler SJ, Martin SW, White PS, Gardiner Q, Lipworth BJ. Evaluation of the importance of head and probe stabilisation in acoustic rhinometry. Rhinology. 2001;39:93-7.

CHAPTER 8
Inflammatory Assessment in Allergic Rhinitis

Antarbhai Patel

■ INTRODUCTION

Rhinitis is a prevalent childhood condition marked by inflammation of the nasal lining. The most common subtype is allergic rhinitis (AR), affecting one out of every six individuals. AR can be categorized into seasonal or perennial types. Previously, AR was thought to be confined to the nose and nasal passages, but recent research indicates that it may be part of a broader systemic airway disease involving the entire respiratory tract. Biopsies from AR patients reveal an accumulation of inflammatory cells, mast cells, and eosinophils in the nasal mucosa. Additionally, there is often an increase in eosinophil granulocytes and eosinophil cationic proteins in the blood. The allergic reactions in AR are attributed to T-helper type 2 lymphocytes, which trigger allergic inflammation and the production of allergen-specific immunoglobulin E. Measuring airway inflammation is crucial for phenotyping AR and asthma. Nitric oxide (NO), a key biological mediator, plays a significant role in the airways by regulating bronchial muscle tone, blood flow, immune response, ciliary movement, and defense mechanisms. Its concentration rises due to eosinophilic inflammation, aiding in diagnosis. Nasal eosinophilia, a characteristic of allergic diseases, also assists in diagnosing and assessing the severity of AR.

■ NITRIC OXIDE

Nitric oxide is an atmospheric pollutant found in vehicle exhaust and cigarette smoke, but it also serves as a biological mediator in both animals and humans. As a biological messenger, NO is crucial in the physiology of various organs and in the pathophysiology of several diseases. In the airways, high levels of the enzyme inducible nitric oxide synthase (NOS2) are expressed in the epithelial cells. Under normal conditions, NO functions as a weak mediator of smooth muscle relaxation, acts as a neurotransmitter in the inhibitory nonadrenergic noncholinergic (iNANC) nervous system, and protects against airway hyperresponsiveness (AHR). Consequently, asthmatics often have elevated NO levels in their exhaled breath, which can serve as an indirect marker for the upregulation of airway inflammation.

LUNG SYNTHESIS OF NITRIC OXIDE

In the lungs, various cell types such as epithelial cells, nerves, vascular endothelial cells, and inflammatory cells can produce NO. L-arginine enters the cells through the cationic amino acid transport (CAT) system and is metabolized by both NO synthases (NOS) and arginases. The airways express three NOS isoforms: (1) Constitutive neural NOS (NOS-I or nNOS), (2) inducible NOS (NOS-II or iNOS), and (3) constitutive endothelial NOS (NOS-III or eNOS). At low concentrations (picomolar range), NO derived from constitutive isoforms in the respiratory tract mediates numerous physiological responses. In contrast, high concentrations of NO (nanomolar range) produced by iNOS are involved in innate immune responses against pathogens and malignant cells, as well as chronic inflammatory diseases. These effects are largely dependent on the reaction between NO and superoxide anion (O_2^-) formed during inflammation, which generates peroxynitrite ($ONOO^-$), a highly reactive oxidant species. Arginases I and II metabolize L-arginine by converting it to L-ornithine, which then synthesizes polyamines and L-proline. Additionally, asymmetric dimethylarginine (ADMA) inhibits NO formation by reducing intracellular L-arginine availability through the arginine/NOS pathway. ADMA competes with L-arginine for binding to NOS, thereby decreasing NO synthesis and increasing the formation of superoxide and peroxynitrite. Consequently, ADMA may facilitate "nitrative-oxidative stress," which leads to protein dysfunction and cellular damage **(Fig. 1)**.

Measurement Technique

Fractional exhaled nitric oxide (FeNO) can be measured using spectroscopic and electroanalytical techniques. Chemiluminescence is the most commonly used spectroscopic method, which involves using a sensitive photomultiplier tube to measure the intensity of fluorescent radiation emitted after the chemical oxidation of NO by ozone. A study by Aerocrine AB in Sweden found a significant correlation, but only moderate agreement, between FeNO values obtained by these two methods, with the electrochemical device recording significantly lower values.

There are two main techniques for estimating exhaled NO. The "online" technique allows the subject to exhale directly into a measurement device **(Figs. 2A to H)**, whereas the "offline" technique involves exhaling into a reservoir that is later connected to the analyzer. In the online method, the person exhales continuously, and the breath is analyzed by an NO analyzer. The NO profile is calculated over time or based on the exhaled volume, along with other exhalation variables such as airway flow rate and pressure.

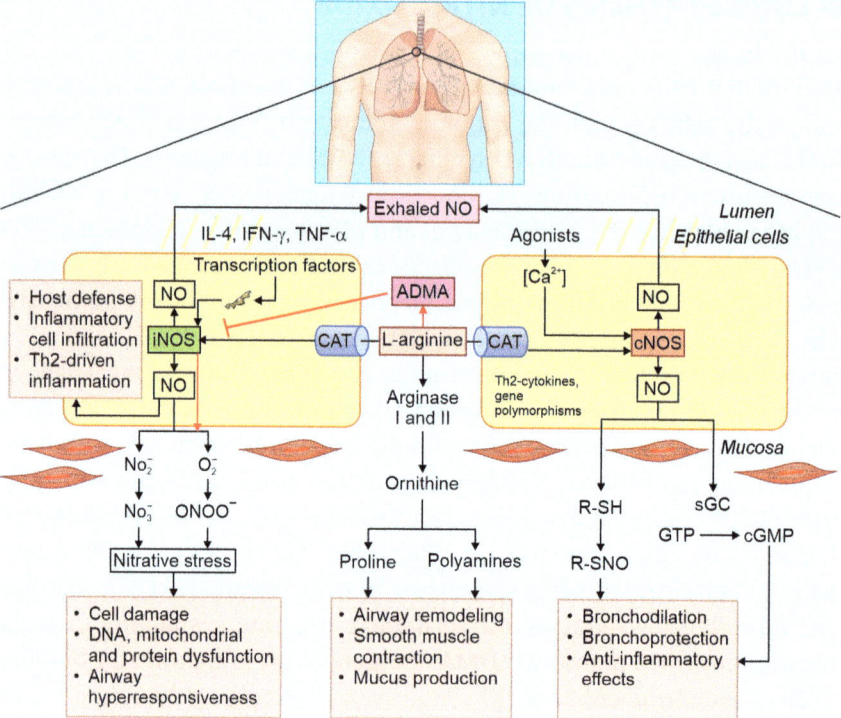

Fig. 1: Schematic representation of nitric oxide (NO) metabolism in the airways. l-Arginine is transported into the cell via the cationic amino acid transport (CAT) system and can be metabolized by both nitric oxide synthases [constitutive NOS (cNOS) and inducible NOS (iNOS)] and arginases (I and II). Moreover, asymmetric dimethylarginine (ADMA), an l-arginine analogue, can competitively inhibit NOS isoforms that, in uncoupling conditions, generate O_2^- and, as consequence, "nitrative stress". (cGMP: cyclic guanosine monophosphate; GTP: guanosine triphosphate; sGC: soluble guanylate cyclase; R-SNO: S-nitrosothiols; R-SH: thiol groups)

Measurement (Fig. 3)

- The single-breath NO profile begins with a washout phase, followed by a plateau of NO.
- Sometimes, the washout phase is followed by an early peak in NO, which may originate from nasal or environmental sources, as well as NO accumulating in the oral and lower airways.
- Early peaks are disregarded, and only the NO plateaus are interpreted.
- The plateau is defined by ensuring sufficient exhalation duration (at least 4 seconds for children under 12 years old and 6 seconds for older children and adults).
- This corresponds to an exhaled volume of at least 0.3 L in adults, assuming an exhalation flow rate of 0.05 L/second.

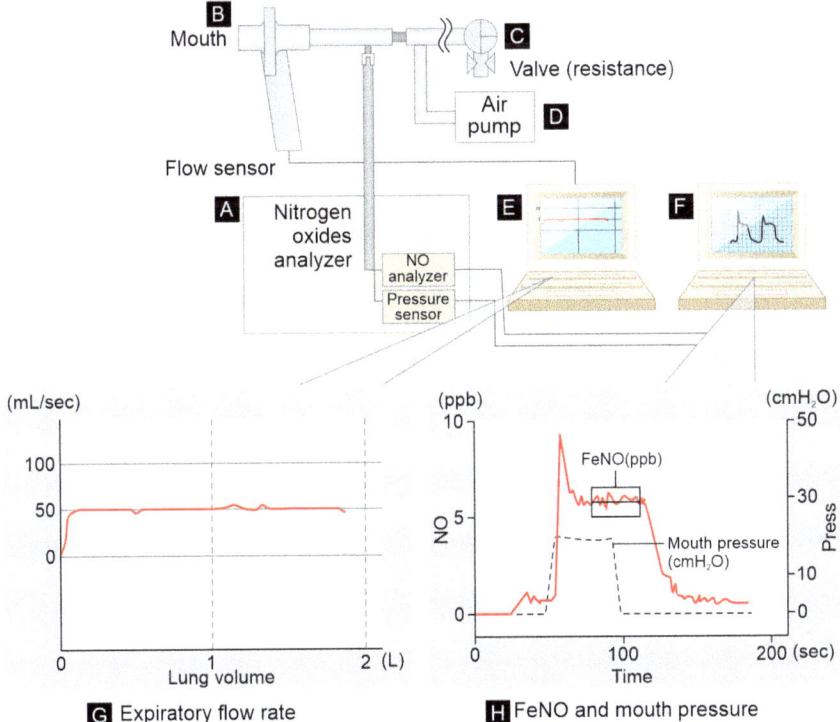

Figs. 2A to H: Fractional exhaled nitric oxide (FeNO) measurement system: (A) Main unit of the measurement device; (B) Expiratory flow-rate sensor; (C) Resistance valve; (D) Air pump; (E) Expiratory flow-rate monitor; (F) FeNO and mouth pressure; (G) Expiratory flow rate; (H) FeNO and mouth pressure.

- The NO plateau concentration is evaluated over a 3-second (0.15 L) window of the exhalation profile.
- The plateau can be flat, positively sloped, or negatively sloped; at least two NO plateau values should agree within 10% of each other.
- Exhaled NO is then calculated as the average of these two values.
- To allow subjects to rest, at least 30 seconds of relaxed tidal breathing off the NO measurement circuit should pass between exhalations.

In adults, there is no correlation between exhaled NO levels and age, whereas in children, FeNO tends to increase with age. Factors such as sex, menstrual cycle, and pregnancy can affect FeNO levels, so these should be documented at the time of measurement. Since spirometry maneuvers temporarily lower exhaled NO levels, it is advised to perform NO analysis before spirometry. FeNO levels can also be influenced by bronchial obstruction, bronchodilators, food, medications, and beverages, so patients should avoid eating and drinking prior to the analysis. Nitrates

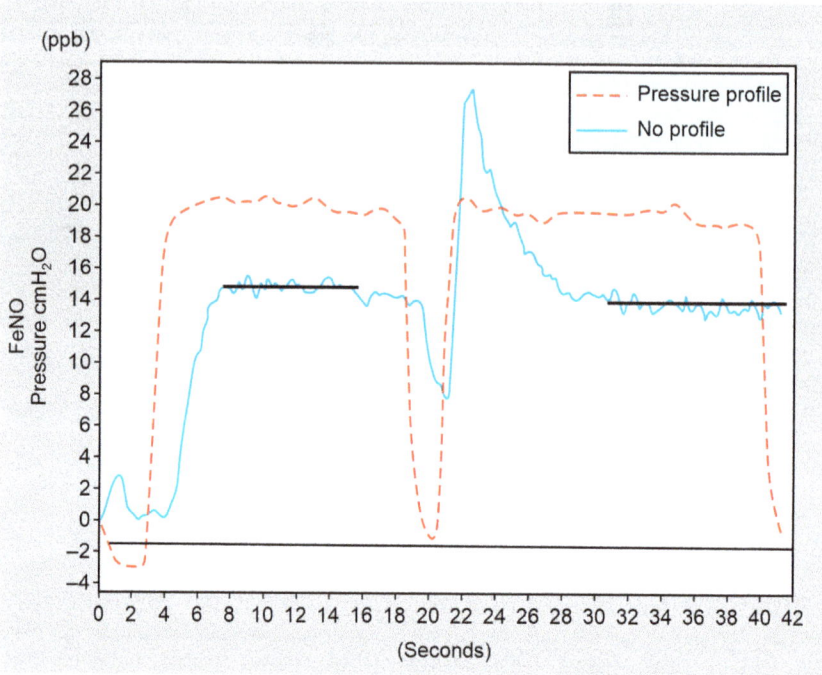

Fig. 3: Differences between the FeNO profiles for air inspired from the oral cavity and the nasal cavity. The vertical axis displays the FeNO or airway pressure over time (horizontal axis). The values for air inspired through the oral cavity are shown on the left side, while the same for the nasal cavity of the same subject are shown on the right side. Due to the high nasal cavity concentrations, NO flows into, and accumulates in, the airways when air is inspired through the nose, forming an initial peak when exhalation starts. However, in the latter half of the expiration, FeNO reaches a plateau with the same value with the initial peak, and therefore, the plateau is reproducible. (FeNO: fractional exhaled nitric oxide; NO: nitric oxide)

and nitrate-rich foods such as lettuce can increase FeNO, while water and caffeine consumption can transiently alter FeNO levels. Alcohol intake reduces FeNO in both asthma patients and healthy individuals. Exhaled NO decreases following treatment with inhaled or oral corticosteroids and inhaled NOS inhibitors. NO levels follow a circadian rhythm, being higher in cases of nocturnal asthma. Chronic smokers exhibit reduced FeNO levels and should abstain from smoking for at least an hour before measurements. Upper and lower respiratory tract viral infections can raise exhaled NO levels in asthma patients, whereas human immunodeficiency virus (HIV) infection is associated with lower exhaled NO levels. Hypoxia also decreases exhaled NO levels. Factors affecting FeNO levels have been described in **Table 1**.

TABLE 1: Influence of various factors on exhaled NO values.	
Increased FeNO	**Decreased FeNO**
Age and height	Females
Males	Smoking
Ethnicity (Chinese)	Lower airway caliber
Viral infections	Alcohol
Nitrates and containing foods (lettuce)	Noneosinophilic asthma
During night	ICS or OCS
	Obesity
	Hypoxia
	HIV infection
	Cystic fibrosis
	Primary ciliary dyskinesia
	Vocal cord dysfunction
	Bronchiectasis
	COPD

(COPD: chronic obstructive pulmonary disease; FeNO: fractional exhaled nitric oxide; HIV: human immunodeficiency virus; ICS: inhaled corticosteroid; NO: nitric oxide; OCS: oral corticosteroid)

REFERENCE FeNO VALUES AND FACTORS AFFECTING FeNO

Numerous studies have been conducted to establish reference values for FeNO in both adults and children, considering the common factors influencing its levels. Based on population studies, key determinants of FeNO values include nonasthmatic status and demographic factors such as age, height, and gender, as well as factors such as viral infections and cigarette smoking. Travers' study on healthy adults found that FeNO levels are significantly affected by atopy, smoking status (current and past), and gender. For example, the highest "upper limit of normal" was observed in atopic males who had never smoked (56.5 ppb), while the lowest was in nonatopic smoking females (30.5 ppb). Another study on healthy nonsmoking individuals identified age and height as key factors, with older and taller subjects having higher FeNO levels. The "upper limit of normal" ranged from 24 ppb (age 25-34 years; height <160 cm) to 54 ppb (age 65-75 years; height >190 cm). A study on healthy children showed FeNO increases with age, with a mean FeNO value of 9.7 ppb and an upper 95% confidence interval (CI) of 25.2 ppb, ranging from 15 ppb at 4 years old to 22.4 ppb at 14–17 years old. Ethnicity also emerged as a significant factor with Chinese children having higher FeNO levels compared to Caucasians. The relationship between age and obesity in adults remains controversial, though several studies indicate higher FeNO levels in men. Increased FeNO levels are positively associated with atopy and viral infections, while both current and previous smoking, as well as passive smoke exposure, tend to lower FeNO levels. FeNO levels are generally lower in cases of smaller airway diameter. Women typically have lower FeNO levels compared to matched men, likely due to the smaller geometry of their airways. FeNO levels may decrease during bronchoconstriction, possibly because of increased airflow velocity in constricted airways when the exhalation rate is kept constant.

■ FRACTIONAL EXHALED NITRIC OXIDE IN RHINITIS

Allergic rhinitis is a significant risk factor for the onset and worsening of asthma. Studies have shown that FeNO levels are elevated in urban non-asthmatic children with atopy compared to nonatopic children, and in children with rhinitis compared to those without rhinitis. This suggests that both atopy and rhinitis can influence FeNO levels. AR has been found to increase FeNO levels compared to atopic controls without rhinitis, but the combination of asthma and AR does not further enhance FeNO levels. This indicates that AR alone can modulate NO production in the lower airways, supporting the "united airways" concept. Chronic rhinosinusitis (CRS), another confounding factor, also increases FeNO levels independently of atopy. CRS patients with lower respiratory symptoms, with or without asthma-like symptoms, show higher FeNO levels compared to those with only rhinitis symptoms, suggesting that CRS can contribute to iNOS-induced lower airway inflammation.

Patients with CRS can be categorized based on eosinophilic and noneosinophilic inflammation of the paranasal sinus mucosa. Eosinophilic CRS patients have higher FeNO levels compared to noneosinophilic CRS patients and normal subjects, indicating that eosinophilic inflammation in the paranasal sinuses affects NO production in the lower airways. A pediatric study found that in children with AR, FeNO is negatively correlated with PD20 methacholine ($r = -0.61$), meaning higher FeNO values are associated with more severe bronchial hyperresponsiveness (BHR). A FeNO cut-off of 32 ppb was predictive of BHR. Similarly, a negative correlation between FeNO levels and BHR severity ($r = -0.58$) was found in adults, with a cut-off of 37 ppb being the best predictor for BHR in AR patients, showing 90.5% specificity, 79.1% sensitivity, and an AUC of 0.90. Detailed interpretation of FeNO values has been described in **Table 2**.

TABLE 2: FeNO values and interpretation.

Interpretation	Adults	Children
Low FeNO	<25 ppb	<20 ppb
Intermediate FeNO	25–50 ppb	20–35 ppb
High FeNO	>50 ppb	>35 ppb
Monitoring	FeNO over 50 ppb	FeNO lower than 50 ppb
Significant increase	>20% increase from base line	>10 ppb absolute increase
Significant response to bronchodilators	>20% decrease from base line	>10 ppb absolute decrease

(FeNO: fractional exhaled nitric oxide)

These findings suggest that FeNO could be a useful predictive marker for BHR in AR patients, aiding in the identification of those at risk for developing asthma. A study by Skiepko et al. found increased FeNO levels in AR patients with BHR during pollen season, with a correlation between increased BHR to histamine and higher FeNO. Another study noted significantly higher FeNO levels in young adults with AR, regardless of the presence of asthma, compared to nonallergic rhinitis subjects. Additionally, perennial sensitization resulted in higher FeNO levels than seasonal sensitization. There was a strong correlation between FeNO and ΔFEV1 after bronchodilation (BD) testing, with FeNO values >34 ppb predicting bronchial reversibility [odds ratio (OR) 1.9], suggesting that FeNO can predict positive BD in AR children.

Finally, it was shown that a body mass index (BMI) value >25 is a risk factor (OR 1.96) for high FeNO levels in AR patients, indicating that overweight status affects FeNO levels. While there is no consensus on the cutoff value for nasal FeNO, an increasing trend in FeNO levels can help manage AR patients.

FRACTIONAL EXHALED NITRIC OXIDE AND PULMONARY FUNCTION

Measuring lung function through spirometry is essential for asthma management. Initially, there was concern that forced respiration during spirometry could influence FeNO results. However, studies have shown that FeNO values in both children and adults are unaffected by prior spirometry if FeNO measurements are taken 10 minutes after baseline spirometry or spirometry conducted pre- and postbronchodilators. Even though repeated spirometry may have an immediate impact on FeNO levels, a 10-minute interval appears to be sufficient for FeNO values to return to prespirometry levels. A study on a pediatric cohort with asthma or AR demonstrated that FeNO levels were strongly correlated with the response to BD testing and could predict bronchial reversibility. This suggests that a simple FeNO measurement can provide valuable information about bronchial reversibility.

■ USE OF FRACTIONAL EXHALED NITRIC OXIDE

- Detect eosinophilic inflammation in the airways.
- Confirm the presence of asthma when objective evidence is required.
- Evaluate corticosteroid effectiveness in people with long-term respiratory symptoms.
- Measure FeNO to guide adjustments in inhaled corticosteroid (ICS) therapy.
- Use FeNO levels to predict asthma relapse following discontinuation of ICS (FeNO levels >49 ppb 4 weeks after stopping steroids).

■ NASAL EOSINOPHILIA

In AR, inflammation of the nasal mucosa is marked by an increase in eosinophils, along with neutrophils, mononuclear cells, and basophils migrating into the nasal tissue during the late-phase allergic reaction. This influx typically peaks 6–12 hours after exposure to an allergen, a response believed to contribute to the chronic nature of the condition. Evaluating eosinophil levels in nasal secretions was suggested as a method to assess eosinophilic inflammation in AR patients, but its diagnostic reliability is limited due to variability influenced by investigator experience and procedural technique.

The technique for collecting nasal eosinophils involves scraping the medial surface of the inferior turbinate with a sterile saline-soaked swab stick. The collected secretions are then evenly spread onto two glass slides, air-dried, fixed with 95% alcohol, and stained with May–Grunwald Giemsa stain. Alternatively, samples can be collected using Merocel sponges placed in the nasal cavity for 10 minutes, followed by centrifugation. The slides are examined under high-power microscopy fields. Interpretation of nasal eosinophils has been described in **Table 3**. Nasal smear analysis is cost-effective, objective, and straightforward, and it finds utility in diagnosing conditions such as nonallergic rhinitis with eosinophilia syndrome (NARES) and in phenotyping CRS.

TABLE 3: Interpretation of eosinophils on nasal smear.

Eosinophils in nasal smear (%)	Description
<5	No eosinophilia
5 to <10	Slight eosinophilia
10 to <50	Moderate eosinophilia
≥50	Marked eosinophilia

CHAPTER 8: Inflammatory Assessment in Allergic Rhinitis

■ SUMMARY

- FeNO serves as a noninvasive marker for detecting eosinophilic inflammation in the airways.
- Tracking serial FeNO levels aids in monitoring treatment responses.
- Elevated eosinophils in nasal secretions assist in diagnosing AR.

■ KEY POINTS

- FeNO serves as a noninvasive marker for detecting eosinophilic inflammation in the airways.
- Cutoff values are not defined in AR.
- Comorbidities and risk factors should be taken into account while interpreting FeNo values.
- Tracking serial FeNO levels aids in monitoring treatment responses.
- Elevated eosinophils in nasal secretions assist phenotype and severity of AR.

■ SUGGESTED READING

1. Amin KAM. Allergic respiratory inflammation and remodeling. Turk Thorac J. 2015;16(3):133-40.
2. Benson VS, Hartl S, Barnes N, Galwey N, Van Dyke MK, Kwon N. Blood eosinophil counts in the general population and airways disease: a comprehensive review and meta-analysis. Eur Respir J. 2022;59(1):2004590.
3. Chakraborty S, Hammar KS, Filiou AE, Holmdahl I, Hoyer A, Ekoff H, et al. Longitudinal eosinophil-derived neurotoxin measurements and asthma development in preschool wheezers. Clin Exp Allergy. 2022;52(11):1338-42.
4. Ciprandi G, Ricciardolo FLM, Signori A, Schiavetti I, Monardo M, Ferraro MR, et al. Increased body mass index and bronchial impairment in allergic rhinitis. Am J Rhinol Allergy. 2013;27:195-201.
5. Ciprandi G, Tosca MA, Capasso M. High exhaled nitric oxide levels may predict bronchial reversibility in allergic children with asthma or rhinitis. J Asthma. 2013;50:33-8.
6. Cirillo I, Ricciardolo F, Medusei G, Signori A, Ciprandi G. Exhaled nitric oxide may predict bronchial hyperreactivity in patients with allergic rhinitis. Int Arch Allergy Immunol. 2013;160:322-8.
7. Global Strategy for Asthma Management and Prevention. Global Initiative for Asthma (GINA). NHLBI/WHO workshop report. Bethesda: National Heart, Lung and Blood Institute; 2014. Avail- able from www.ginasthma.org/ [updated].
8. Granger V, Zerimech F, Arab J, Siroux V, de Nadai P, Tsicopoulos A, et al. Blood eosinophil cationic protein and eosinophil-derived neurotoxin are associated with different asthma expression and evolution in adults. Thorax. 2022;77(6):552-562.
9. Haccuria A, Michils A, Michiels S, Van Muylem A. Exhaled nitric oxide: a biomarker integrating both lung function and airway inflammation changes. J Allergy Clin Immunol. 2014;134:554-9.

10. Hanania NA, Wenzel S, Rosén K, Hsieh HJ, Mosesova S, Choy DF, et al. Exploring the effects of omalizumab in allergic asthma: an analysis of biomarkers in the EXTRA study. Am J Respir Crit Care Med. 2013;187:804-11.
11. Harter K, Hammel G, Krabiell L, Linkohr B, Peters A, Schwettmann L, et al. Different Psychosocial Factors Are Associated with Seasonal and Perennial Allergies in Adults: Cross-Sectional Results of the KORA FF4 Study. Int Arch Allergy Immunol. 2019;179(4):262-72.
12. Holguin F, Comhair SA, Hazen SL, Powers RW, Khatri SS, Bleecker ER, et al. An association between l-arginine/asymmetric dimethyl arginine balance, obesity, and the age of asthma onset phenotype. Am J Respir Crit Care Med. 2013;187:153-9.
13. Honkoop PJ, Loijmans RJ, Termeer EH, Snoeck-Stroband JB, van den Hout WB, Bakker MJ, et al. Symptom- and fraction of exhaled nitric oxide-driven strategies for asthma control: a cluster-randomized trial in primary care. J Allergy Clin Immunol. 2014.
14. Kakli HA, Riley TD. Allergic Rhinitis. Prim Care. 2016;43(3):465-75.
15. Mahr TA, Malka J, Spahn JD. Inflammometry in pediatric asthma: a review of fractional exhaled nitric oxide in clinical practice. Allergy Asthma Proc. 2013;34:210-9.
16. Malerba M, Ragnoli B, Radaeli A, Ricciardolo FLM. Long-term adjustment of stable asthma treatment with fractional exhaled nitric oxide and sputum eosinophils. Eur J Inflamm. 2012;10:383-92.
17. Petsky HL, Cates CJ, Lasserson TJ, Li AM, Turner C, Kynaston JA, et al. A systematic review and meta-analysis: tailoring asthma treatment on eosinophilic markers (exhaled nitric oxide or sputum eosinophils). Thorax. 2012;67:199-208.
18. Ricciardolo FL, Di Stefano A, Silvestri M, Van Schadewijk AM, Malerba M, Hiemstra PS, et al. Exhaled nitric oxide is related to bronchial eosinophilia and airway hyperresponsiveness to bradykinin in allergen-induced asthma exacerbation. Int J Immunopathol Pharmacol. 2012;25:175-82.
19. Small P, Keith PK, Kim H. Allergic rhinitis. Allergy Asthma Clin Immunol. 2018;14(Suppl 2):51.
20. Syk J, Malinovschi A, Johansson G, Undén AL, Andreasson A, Lekander M, et al. Anti-inflammatory treatment of atopic asthma guided by exhaled nitric oxide: a randomized, controlled trial. J Allergy Clin Immunol Pract. 2013;1:639-48.
21. Takeno S, Taruya T, Ueda T, Noda N, Hirakawa K. Increased exhaled nitric oxide and its oxidation metabolism in eosinophilic chronic rhinosinusitis. Auris Nasus Larynx. 2013;40:458-64.
22. Tsuda T, Maeda Y, Nishide M, Koyama S, Hayama Y, Nojima S et al. Eosinophil-derived neurotoxin enhances airway remodeling in eosinophilic chronic rhinosinusitis and correlates with disease severity. Int Immunol. 2019;31(1):33-40.
23. Verbanck S, Kerckx Y, Schuermans D, Vincken W, Paiva M, Van Muylem A. Effect of airways constriction on exhaled nitric oxide. J Appl Physiol (1985). 2008;104:925-30.

CHAPTER 9

Allergy Tests

*Taha A Qureshi, Tabasum Shafi, Ayaz Gull,
Aabid M Koul, Muzima Jeelani, Roohi Rasool*

■ INTRODUCTION

Among various allergic diseases, allergic rhinitis (AR) represents a significant global health burden, affecting millions of individuals worldwide. The accurate diagnosis of such conditions is therefore essential for effective management and improved patient outcomes. To this end, various investigations are available, each offering unique insights into the underlying immune mechanisms and allergen sensitivities. This chapter provides a thorough appraisal of the most frequently used diagnostic tests in allergy, both in vivo and in vitro.

■ IN VIVO ALLERGY TESTS

In vivo allergy tests are diagnostic procedures that involve exposing the body to allergens to observe and assess the resulting allergic reactions. These tests are conducted directly on or within the body and are typically performed in clinical settings under the supervision of healthcare professionals. In vivo testing is invaluable in identifying specific allergens responsible for triggering allergic reactions in individuals and offer several advantages, including immediate results, relatively low cost, and the ability to assess allergic reactions in real-time. However, they also have limitations, such as the potential for false-positive or false-negative results, variability in interpretation between healthcare providers, and the risk of inducing allergic reactions in sensitive individuals. It is for these reasons important to carry out such procedures in a controlled set-up where any untoward reaction can be handled. Despite few of these limitations, in vivo allergy tests remain a crucial component of the diagnostic process for AR.

Skin Prick Test

Skin prick test (SPT) by far is considered as the gold standard and the most reliable approach in delineating the immunoglobulin E (IgE)-mediated underlying mechanism in AR. It is rapid, safe, and cost-effective office-based procedure for detecting clinically relevant allergens. The test interpretation relies on the presence and degree of cutaneous reactivity as a surrogate marker for allergen sensitization. Through the introduction of relevant allergens onto the skin surface, a cascade is initiated leading to the cross-linking of specific IgE (sIgE) bound to the surface receptors on mast cells, subsequently leading to their degranulation and the release of histamine along with other mediators. These mediators, in turn, exert their effects on the skin, eliciting a distinct wheal and flare response. The quantification of this response enables clinicians to arrive at a specific diagnosis. Such precision facilitates the development of tailored treatment modalities, including allergen avoidance strategies and immunotherapy, based on individual sensitization profiles.

Multiple and various classes of allergens can be tested at the same time since the resulting reaction to the particular allergen is mostly restricted to the immediate vicinity of the SPT. It was Lewis and Grant in 1926 who first described SPT, albeit further credit goes to Jack Pepys who in 1970s got it perfected and popularized. SPT is minimally invasive, carries the advantage of being cost-friendly to the patient, and the results are quickly available in just 15–20 minutes. Moreover, the results are reproducible provided the procedure is carried out by well-trained health professionals. The test gives visual satisfaction and reinforces the belief about the sensitivity in the patient which is very useful in impacting the patient's behavior viz-à-viz his compliance to the management plan.

Selection of Antigens for Skin Prick Test

For an optimal selection of the testing panel of inhalant allergens especially pollens, the knowledge about the local aerobiological data is extremely important. A general cross-reactivity among the botanical families obviates the need to include a large number of cross-reacting allergens. Just one or two locally important representatives from each group is good enough. Inhalant allergens used for diagnosis of AR will enlist:
- *Indoor allergens:* House dust mites, animal dander (cats and dogs), insects (especially cockroach), and fungi.
- *Outdoor allergens:* Grass, weed, tree pollens, and fungal spores.

Skin Prick Testing Procedure

After obtaining a written informed consent, a drop of the antigen extract is placed on the skin and a lancet is passed through the drop to penetrate the skin at around an angle of 45°. A small break in the epidermis is created by gently lifting the device **(Fig. 1)**. A general estimate is that approximately 3 µL of fluid get into the skin. To ensure standardization, histamine and normal saline will be used as positive and negative controls respectively. Saline, the negative control, signifies the baseline reactivity of the skin. The histamine-positive control is used to rule out any interference by an agent that suppresses the skin reactivity. For the skin test results to be valid, the

CHAPTER 9: Allergy Tests

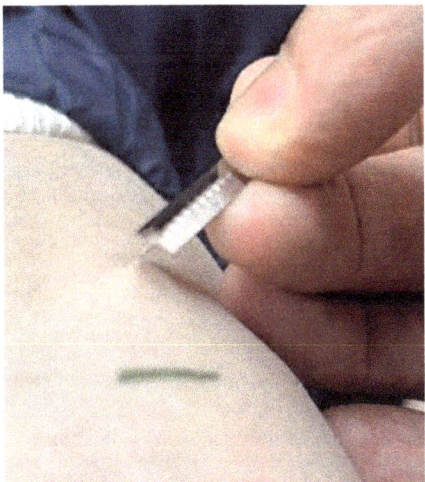

Fig. 1: Skin prick test.
Courtesy: Ayaz Gull.

wheal diameter of the negative control has to be <3 mm in diameter while as the wheal size at the histamine pricking site has to be 3 mm or more than the wheal at the negative control site. In case the wheal at the histamine site is <3 mm, it suggests some interference such as suppression by antihistamines. The patient, before the test, therefore has to be off the antihistaminic, immune-suppressants, and the like for varied periods before testing to avoid any such interference with the skin response **(Table 1)**. Saline is pricked first, followed by allergens and histamine at the last.

Interpretation

At 20 minutes after pricking, if the wheal diameter is 3 mm or more than that of the negative control, the test result is read as positive while less than that is read as negative **(Fig. 2)**. The antigens whose result comes positive, the patient is reported as sensitized to those, and a second history is taken to verify the clinical correlation and thereby the subsequent specific and customized management of the patient with AR.

Sensitivity and Specificity of Skin Prick Test

In terms of identifying individuals with or without allergic reactions, specificity and sensitivity are crucial factors in the SPT that can impact the precision of allergen detection. A highly specific test means that false-positive results are unlikely. When it comes to the SPT, specificity can differ based on factors such as the allergen being tested and the use of appropriate controls. Research indicates that the SPT generally has a high specificity, often >90% for prevalent

TABLE 1: Abstinence period of various drugs prior to skin prick test.

Drug	Abstinence before testing
First-generation short-acting H1 blocker antihistamines: Pheniramine, chlorpheniramine, promethazine, diphenhydramine, dimenhydrinate, carbinoxamine, clemastine, mepyramine, dimethindene, cinnarizine, meclizine, and cyclizine	3 days
First-generation long-action H1 blockers: Hydroxyzine and brompheniramine	7 days
Second-generation long-acting H1 blockers: Cetirizine, loratadine, desloratadine, levocetirizine, ebastine, mizolastine, and bepotastine	7 days
Second-generation long-acting H1 blockers: Fexofenadine and dexchlorpheniramine	5 days
Second-generation short-acting H1 blockers: Azelastine and olopatadine	3 days
H1 blocker: Cyproheptadine	14 days
H1 blocker: Ketotifen	14 days
Topical steriods on skin	21 days
Topical antihistamine ointment or cream	7 days
Intranasal steroids and intranasal or intraocular cromoglycate and nedocromil	0
Inhaled steroids	0
Depot steroid such as Kenacort and Depo-Medrol	90 days
Short-term oral prednisolone or equivalent 30 mg/day for 5–7 days	0
Short-term oral steroids, prednisolone or equivalent >40 mg/day for 7 days or more	10 days
Systematic/long-term steroids, prednisolone or equivalent >10 mg/day for >10 days	10 days
Topical calcineurin inhibitors such as tacrolimus	7 days
Other systematic drugs: Omalizumab	6 months
Leukotriene receptor antagonist such as montelukast and zafirlukast	0
Cyclosporine A	0
Theophylline	0
Tricyclic antidepressants: Amitriptyline, amoxapine, desipramine, doxepin, imipramine, nortriptyline, protriptyline, and trimipramine	14 days

Contd...

Contd...

Drug	Abstinence before testing
Tranquilizers: Benzodiazepines such as alprazolam, clobazam, clonazepam, clorazepate, chlordiazepoxide, diazepam, estazolam, lorazepam, oxazepam, temazepam, and triazolam	7 days
Inhaled bronchodilators such as salbutamol, salmeterol, bambuterol, terbutaline, formoterol, and levosalbutamol	0
Phenothiazines: Chlorpromazine, fluphenazine, mesoridazine, perphenazine, prochlorperazine, promazine, thioridazine, trifluoperazine, and triflupromazine	7 days
Selective serotonin reuptake inhibitors (SSRIs): Citalopram, escitalopram, paroxetine, fluoxetine, fluvoxamine, and sertraline	0
Long-acting oral and parenteral bronchodilators	24 hours
Intranasal and intraocular antihistamine such as olopatadine and azelastine	2 days
Ayurveda, homeopathy, unani, herbal and such medicines with label	7 days
Ayurveda, homeopathy, unani, herbal, and such medicines without label	28 days
Oral plain bronchodilators	12 hours
Selective norepinephrine reuptake inhibitors (SNRIs) and protein pump inhibitors (PPIs)	0
H2 blockers such as cimetidine, ranitidine, and famotidine	2 days
Alternative medicines such as butterbur, stinging nettle, citrus unshiu powder, *Lycopus lucidus*, spirulina, cellulose powder, traditional Chinese medicine, and Indian herbal products such as tulasi and amruthaballi	7 days

Source: Adapted with permission "Skin Prick test-standards of practice for diagnosis of Allergy."—Pendakur Anand

allergens such as animal epithelia, dust mites, and pollens. On the contrary, sensitivity refers to the test's capacity to accurately detect individuals who have developed sensitivity to an allergen, thus minimizing the chances of false negatives. Particular allergens and individual variances in skin reactions can significantly affect the SPT's sensitivity. Typically, sensitivity to common inhalant allergens range from 70% to 95%. Nevertheless, sensitivity might be reduced for specific allergens, like foods, due to cross-reactivity and variations in allergenic proteins, which can result in inconsistencies in test outcomes. Overall SPTs display significant degrees of sensitivity (79–97%), specificity (80–91%), positive predictive value (PPV) (79–93%), and negative predictive value (NPV) (74–97%) in diagnosing allergies in general.

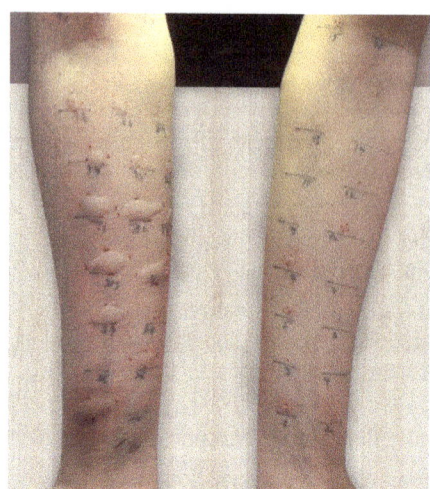

Fig. 2: Wheal and flare responses of skin prick test.
Courtesy: Ayaz Gull.

In general, the SPT's efficacy in allergy diagnosis is underscored by its equilibrium between specificity and sensitivity. Clinicians frequently utilize this invaluable tool for detecting sensitization to specific allergens. However, to enhance the accuracy of diagnosis and overcome limitations in both specificity as well as sensitivity, they often combine it with additional diagnostic procedures such as serum-sIgE testing or oral food challenges. By employing a range of methods, the probability of inaccurate results can be reduced, resulting in improved allergy assessments, therefore eventually enhancing patient outcomes.

Contraindications of Skin Prick Test

- Severe dermatographism, active skin infections, inflammation, or other skin conditions affecting the test site, which may interfere with accurate interpretation.
- Recent use of antihistamines or other medications that can suppress allergic reactions, potentially leading to false-negative results **(Table 1)**.
- Patients with unstable severe asthma. Asthma must be controlled satisfactorily and patient must be stable before the procedure.
- History of anaphylaxis or severe allergic reactions, as SPT may pose a risk of triggering a severe reaction.
- *Pregnancy:* SPT must be considered very carefully in view of a remote possibility of inducing a systemic allergic reaction that could induce uterine contractions if it necessitates the use of epinephrine that is thought to cause constriction of the umbilical artery.

Provocation Tests

The allergen provocation test serves as a well-established model for comprehending allergic airway conditions such as asthma and AR. It enables the assessment of allergen-induced changes in respiratory function and inflammatory processes in sensitized individuals, along with their relationships. In the realm of upper airways, allergen challenge primarily focuses on evaluating the clinical and pathophysiological outcomes of the early allergic response, serving diagnostic and research purposes alike. Additionally, allergen challenge has proven invaluable in exploring the interaction between upper and lower airways and understanding the mechanisms of drug development in proof-of-mechanism studies.

The allergen challenge test has been a key method for diagnosing allergic conditions, providing direct evidence of how specific allergens relate to symptoms and disease severity. While efforts continue to improve standardization, availability, and safety for routine clinical use, many challenge tests have become reliable diagnostic tools used by proficient medical personnel. Although allergen provocation tests are needed less often, they have historical significance tracing back to early methods such as the patch test in 1894.

Nasal Provocation Test

Currently, nasal allergen challenge (NAC) is used in upper airway diagnostics and research, focusing on early allergic responses, symptom evaluation, and acute proinflammatory mediator release. Conversely, while occupational agents are common tools for diagnosing and researching occupational asthma in lower airways, allergen extract challenges are mostly limited to specialized research settings.

Confirming AR is straightforward when atopic sensitization aligns with clinical history, verified by serum-sIgE antibodies or a SPT. However, discrepancies between sensitization and clinical history, or the absence of systemic atopy despite suggestive AR symptoms (referred to as local AR), may necessitate a nasal allergen provocation test (NAPT). Accurate differentiation from nonallergic conditions is crucial for proper management. Occupational allergy (OA) also warrants NAPT when standardized allergens are unavailable for SPT kits or sIgE measurement.

Determining the suitability of allergen-specific immunotherapy (AIT) for AR relies on demonstrating AR symptom induction by allergens, which may not always be evident from patient history, particularly in polysensitized patients. Various NAPT approaches exist, each with advantages and limitations. For routine clinical use, qualitative symptom scale assessments suffice, while research demands quantitative methods with high reproducibility.

Nasal allergen provocation test can elicit immediate, late, dual immediate and late, or delayed responses, with conjunctival responses commonly observed. Washout periods vary depending on sensitization type and previous medication usage.

During the provocation, physician presence and emergency kits are essential to manage potential adverse reactions. Patients should acclimate in the testing room before the challenge, starting with a control solution followed by allergen administration at increasing concentrations, with reactions recorded accordingly. Postchallenge, patients may use local decongestive sprays and/or antihistamines. Various allergen application methods are employed, with nasal spray preferred for precise dosing. Careful monitoring of solution parameters is crucial.

Nasal allergen provocation test is generally safe, even for asthma patients, but improper technique or excessive dosing may trigger bronchoconstriction. Pharyngeal itching is common, while severe reactions are rare.

Conjunctival Allergen Provocation Test

The conjunctival allergen provocation test (CAPT), also known as conjunctival allergen challenge (CAC), involves applying specified concentrations of an allergen solution to the ocular conjunctiva to elicit an IgE-mediated allergic response if the patient is sensitized. It is a systematic test used to assess inflammatory responses on the outer eye surface following allergen administration, primarily to determine reactivity to specific allergens at the mucosal level.

Conjunctival allergen provocation test is valuable for investigating IgE-mediated hypersensitivity disorders affecting the eyes, helping identify or confirm allergens responsible for ocular symptoms and highlighting reactivity patterns. Recently, CAPT has been used as a surrogate test for assessing mucosal reactivity in various allergic conditions, including rhinitis, asthma, food allergies, and latex allergies. Despite being safe, simple, and efficient in evaluating allergic diseases, CAPT is underutilized in routine clinical practice compared to investigative settings.

Procedure: Before starting the test, there is a pretest adjustment period of 15 minutes to prepare the patient. Subjective and objective measurements are taken to establish baseline data. A control formulation is then applied to the outer layer of the eyeball. After 15 minutes, another round of subjective and objective measurements is taken to assess any initial reactions.
1. If a positive reaction occurs at this stage, the test is halted, and appropriate medication is administered immediately. In the absence of a reaction, an allergen is administered into the other eye. After another 15 minutes, measurements are taken again.

2. If a positive reaction occurs after allergen administration, the test is stopped, and medication is given promptly.

Following the completion of the test, the patient is observed for a further 2 hours to monitor for any delayed reactions or complications.

■ IN VITRO ALLERGY TESTS

In vitro allergy testing are diagnostic methods that analyze allergic responses outside of the body, typically in laboratory settings. Unlike in vivo tests, which involve exposing the body to allergens directly, in vitro tests rely on blood samples to detect allergen-specific immune responses. These tests are less invasive and do not require direct exposure to allergens, making them safer and more comfortable for patients, particularly those with severe allergies or skin conditions. Unlike SPT, no curfew on intake of medication is required prior to performing of these tests. However, they are less specific and more costly, limiting their accessibility in some healthcare settings.

Total Immunoglobulin E Test

Immunoglobulin E constitutes a class of antibodies synthesized by plasma cells in response to exposure to allergens. It ranks as the least abundant antibody type, with approximately 50% circulating as free IgE within the intravascular compartment, while the remaining fraction bound to IgE receptors located on various cells, particularly mast cells and basophils, via the high-affinity IgE receptor (FcεRI).

While total immunoglobulin E (total IgE) is a valuable screening tool for predicting AR, it cannot be considered a reliable marker as it provides only gross information, is nonspecific and its levels are also increased in non-allergic conditions, such as parasitic infections, some primary immunodeficiencies, and certain malignancies. Conversely, diminished or standard levels do not exclude the existence of IgE-mediated diseases. Thus, the overall IgE levels necessitate meticulous interpretation and should not be solely relied upon as indicative of allergic conditions.

In the past, quantifying total IgE levels involved utilizing diverse immunoassays that employed specific antibodies targeting human IgE as either capture or detection agents. These antibodies were commonly affixed to a solid phase as capture antibodies or directly labeled with radioisotopes, enzymes, or fluorophores. The advent of automated platforms has significantly improved accuracy and reliability, leading to enhanced specificity and sensitivity in IgE determination.

Specific IgE Test

Total immunoglobulin E has long been utilized as a conventional marker for assessing allergic conditions, yet its specificity is relatively limited and its elevation is not exclusively indicative of allergy. sIgE testing serves as a valuable diagnostic tool by detecting allergen-sIgE antibodies in patients' blood samples. Unlike total IgE measurement, sIgE testing offers allergen-specificity, enabling precise identification of the allergens triggering allergic reactions.

Tests for allergen-sIgE in the blood are used as a second-line option to confirm sensitization to common allergens. These tests are sensitive and have nearly similar diagnostic accuracy to SPT. SPTs require a healthy skin area, patients need to abstain from antihistamine medications and SPTs carry a minimal risk of a systemic reaction. Serum tests, on the other hand, are unaffected by antihistamines or extensive skin conditions.

Various in vitro sIgE testing technologies exist, with fluorescence enzyme immunoassay (FEIA) being the most extensively researched and considered the gold standard for sIgE measurement. In the past, radioallergosorbent tests (RAST) pioneered the detection of serum allergen-specific antibodies. These tests progressed into second-generation semiquantitative IgE assays and further advanced into third-generation automated analyzers, such as ImmunoCAP System (Phadia, Thermo Scientific, Uppsala, Sweden) and Immulite 2000 (Diagnostic Products Corporation, Los Angeles, CA, USA). These modern methods use nonisotopic markers, resulting in faster and more precise analysis with improved accuracy and sensitivity compared to earlier techniques.

The ImmunoCAP FEIA has become a standard method for quantifying sIgE antibodies to a wide range of allergen extracts and their individual molecular components. Introduced as a second-generation immunoassay in 1989, the assay involves sIgE binding to a solid-phase, with allergen components covalently coupled to a capsulated cellulose polymer, followed by the addition of a β-galactosidase-labeled anti-IgE antibody to form an antigen-antibody immune complex. Subsequent fluorescence detection using a fluorogenic substrate correlates the fluorescence signal with the concentration of allergen-bound IgE, as determined from a standard curve. This method offers a robust and reliable means of assessing allergic sensitization profiles with high precision and reproducibility.

Specific IgE measurements encompass two main types of assays: (1) Singleplex and (2) multiplex. Singleplex assays assess IgE antibodies against individual allergens, offering analysis for one allergen at a time. Conversely, multiplex assays allow simultaneous measurement of IgE antibodies against multiple allergens and their individual molecular components within a single test, providing a comprehensive overview of allergic sensitivities. While singleplex assays are commonly used when testing for a limited number of allergens or when there is a known allergen of interest, multiplex assays are advantageous for screening a wide range of allergens simultaneously, reducing the need for multiple tests and offering a comprehensive assessment. The choice between the two depends on factors such as the number of allergens to be tested and clinical requirements.

Component-resolved Diagnostics

Component-resolved diagnostics (CRD) represents a significant advancement in allergy diagnosis by determining sIgE antibodies against multiple individual components of the allergen rather than whole allergen extracts. This approach, also known as molecular diagnostics or multiplex sIgE testing is recommended as one useful option in patients who have uncertain diagnostic outcomes based on their clinical history and whole extract-based IgE allergen tests (SPT or sIgE). CRD has significantly enhanced the accuracy and specificity of allergy diagnostics, leading to more precise diagnosis, better risk assessment, and tailored AIT.

In the context of AR, the indications of carrying out CRD are the same as that for FEIA. Moreover, CRD testing is useful particularly for those patients with concurrent respiratory and food allergies. In circumstances where there is a strong indication for AIT but a confusing picture of oligo or polysensitization to inhalant allergens is confronted, CRD may enhance the accuracy of allergy diagnosis.

Allergens and Their Components

Allergen sources, such as pollen, house dust mite, peanut, and hymenoptera typically consist of various allergenic parts known as allergen components that contain distinct epitopes, which are specific three-dimensional binding sites for corresponding IgE antibodies. Cross-reactivity occurs when epitopes in different allergen sources resemble each other, leading to allergic reactions to multiple allergens.

Allergen sources are named according to their Latin family names, such as *Arachis hypogaea* for peanuts. Each allergen source contains multiple allergen components, typically identified by numbers, e.g., *Ara h1* represents allergen number 1 from *A. hypogaea*. Some common allergens and their common allergenic components are depicted in **Table 2**.

Advantages

One of the primary benefits of CRD is its ability to differentiate between "genuine" and "cross-reactive" components in individuals with polysensitization, a level of resolution unattainable with conventional testing methods. Implementing CRD in such cases not only enhances diagnostic precision but also guides the appropriate administration of allergy immunotherapy, as treatment responses vary based on the determination of genuine or cross-reactive allergen sensitization. CRD also facilitates the

TABLE 2: Some common allergens and some of their allergenic components.

Common allergen	Latin name	Allergenic components
House dust mites	Dermatophagoides pteronyssinus, Dermatophagoides farina	Der p 1, Der p 2, Der p 23, Der f 1, Der f 2
Pollen (grasses)	Poaceae family	Phl p 1, Phl p 2, Phl p 5, Phl p 6
Pollen (trees)	Various	Birch (Bet v 1, Bet v 2, Bet v 4)
Pollen (weeds)	Various	Ragweed (Amb a 1), Mugwort (Art v 1), English plantain (Pla l 1), Pellitory (Par j 2)
Cat	Felis domesticus	Fel d 1, Fel d 2, Fel d 4, Fel d 7, Fel d 8
Dog	Canis lupus familiaris	Can f 1, Can f 2, Can f 4
Cockroach	Blattella germanica	Bla g 1, Bla g 2, Bla g 4, Bla g 5
Peanut	Arachis hypogaea	Ara h 1, Ara h 2, Ara h 3, Ara h 6, Ara h 8
Tree nuts	Various	Almond (Pru du 6), Cashew (Ana o 3), Walnut (Jug r 1)
Egg	Gallus gallus domesticus	Gal d 1, Gal d 2, Gal d 3, Gal d 4, Gal d 5
Cow milk	Bos taurus	Bos d 4, Bos d 5, Bos d 6, Bos d 8, Bos d 9
Wheat	Triticum aestivum	Tri a 14, Tri a 19, Tri a 21, Tri a 28, Tri a 36
Soy	Glycine max	Gly m 4, Gly m 5, Gly m 6, Gly m 8
Fish	Various	Cod (Gad c 1), Salmon (Sal s 1), Tuna (Thu a, Thu a 1)
Latex	Hevea brasiliensis	Hev b 1, Hev b 3, Hev b 5, Hev b 6.02, Hev b 11
Mold	Aspergillus, Alternaria, Cladosporium	Alt a 1, Cla h 2, Asp f 1, Asp f 3, Asp f 6

determination of genuine coreactivity and cross-reactivity, particularly crucial in complex cases where patients exhibit sIgE reactivity against numerous antigens. In addition, CRD offers a significant advantage in differentiating between allergenic components such as ovomucoid and ovalbumin, in cases of egg allergy. This level of specificity is crucial as ovomucoid is more heat-stable than ovalbumin, and individuals allergic to ovomucoid may experience reactions to both cooked and raw egg, whereas those allergic to ovalbumin might only react to raw egg. Therefore, CRD aids in personalized management strategies by minimizing unnecessary dietary restrictions and reducing the risk of accidental exposure to allergens.

Limitations

While CRD allows for testing sIgE against multiple allergen components, surpassing the capacity of prick testing, some diagnostic challenges persist for certain patients. Studies suggest that while CRD may offer enhanced specificity, it often lacks sensitivity compared to standard skin prick testing and sIgE level measurements. Nonetheless, CRD detects a broader range of allergens than prick testing and sIgE measurements, making it a valuable tool when these standard diagnostic tests yield inconclusive results.

INTERPRETING ALLERGY TEST FINDINGS: A COMPREHENSIVE APPROACH

Interpreting allergy test results, whether obtained through blood or skin testing, requires consideration of various factors including the patient's clinical symptoms, age, relevant allergen exposures, and the sensitivity, specificity, and reproducibility of the test used. It is important to note that the detection of allergen-sIgE indicates sensitization rather than allergy itself. Therefore, a positive sIgE result in the absence of allergic symptoms or a negative response to allergen exposure should be deemed clinically irrelevant. Many children with positive test results may not exhibit any clinical symptoms upon allergen exposure. This underscores the importance for clinicians to gather detailed medical histories and understand the characteristics of specific illnesses when selecting and interpreting allergy tests. Testing for a wide range of allergens without considering factors such as medical history, geographic relevance, and disease characteristics may lead to numerous clinically irrelevant positive results. Overinterpretation of these results could result in unnecessary allergen avoidance measures, which may have negative social, emotional, and/or nutritional consequences. Similarly, caution is warranted when test results are negative despite a convincing medical history of allergy.

SUMMARY

For the diagnosis of type I IgE-mediated allergic diseases, SPTs remain the primary method to detect allergen-sIgE antibodies bound to mast cells on the skin surface of sensitized individuals. This approach is the gold standard and yields reliable results. Besides, serum IgE detection in vitro using highly purified allergens or recombinant molecules, either individually or in multiplex formats, serves as a complementary or alternative diagnostic method. Serum IgE testing poses minimal risk to patients, involving only a blood sample, and is preferred in cases of high risk of anaphylaxis, interference from essential medications, young age, or limited skin availability due to skin conditions. In addition to skin and serum IgE tests, provocation tests may also be employed in certain cases to confirm allergic reactions. However, provocation tests carry inherent risks and are typically reserved for situations where other diagnostic methods are inconclusive or impractical.

■ KEY POINTS

- Allergic rhinitis is a significant global health concern, highlighting the importance of precise diagnostic methods.
- In vivo allergy tests, such as SPT and provocation tests, conducted directly on the body to observe allergic reactions are specific, offer immediate results, and are relatively cost-effective.
- In vitro allergy tests, encompassing total IgE measurement, sIgE assays, and CRD, do not require direct exposure to allergens and are particularly beneficial for patients with severe allergies or skin conditions.
- Test interpretation of both in vivo and in vitro allergy tests requires careful consideration of various factors such as clinical history, symptoms, and test results to arrive at an accurate diagnosis and guide appropriate management strategies.

■ SUGGESTED READING

1. Ansotegui IJ, Melioli G, Canonica GW, Caraballo L, Villa E, Ebisawa M, et al. IgE allergy diagnostics and other relevant tests in allergy, a World Allergy Organization position paper. World Allergy Organ J. 2020;13(2):100080. Erratum in: World Allergy Organ J. 2021;14(7):100557.
2. Augé J, Vent J, Agache I, Airaksinen L, Campo Mozo P, Chaker A, et al. EAACI Position paper on the standardization of nasal allergen challenges. Allergy. 2018;73(8):1597-608.
3. Callery EL, Keymer C, Barnes NA, Rowbottom AW. Component-resolved diagnostics in the clinical and laboratory investigation of allergy. Ann Clin Biochem. 2020;57(1):26-35.
4. Kwong KY, Eghrari-Sabet JS, Mendoza GR, Platts-Mills T, Horn R. The benefits of specific immunoglobulin E testing in the primary care setting. Am J Manag Care. 2011;17 Suppl 17:S447-59.
5. Luengo O, Cardona V. Component resolved diagnosis: when should it be used? Clin Transl Allergy. 2014;4:28.
6. Melillo G, Bonini S, Cocco G, Davies RJ, de Monchy JG, Frølund L, et al. EAACI provocation tests with allergens. Report prepared by the European Academy of Allergology and Clinical Immunology Subcommittee on provocation tests with allergens. Allergy. 1997;52(35 Suppl):1-35.
7. Qureshi TA, Qadri Q, Shafi T, Shah ZA, Kundangar A, Rasool R. Pre skin prick testing: a curfew required on herbals too. J Cell Immunother. 2018;4(2):83-6.
8. San Miguel-Rodríguez A, Armentia A, Martín-Armentia S, Martín-Armentia B, Corell A, Lozano-Estevan MC, et al. Component-resolved diagnosis in allergic disease: Utility and limitations. Clin Chim Acta. 2019;489:219-24.
9. Scadding G, Hellings P, Alobid I, Bachert C, Fokkens W, van Wijk RG, et al. Diagnostic tools in Rhinology EAACI position paper. Clin Transl Allergy. 2011;1(1):2.
10. Sicherer SH, Wood RA; American Academy of Pediatrics Section On Allergy And Immunology. Allergy testing in childhood: using allergen-specific IgE tests. Pediatrics. 2012;129(1):193-7.

SECTION 3

Therapeutics

Section Editor: Kasyapi Nagaraju

- **Controllers**
  Shebna A Khader

- **Preventers**
  Samyugtha

- **Disease Modifiers**
  R Prasanna

- **Surgical Intervention in Allergic Rhinitis**
  Deepak Kumar

CHAPTER 10

Controllers

Shebna A Khader

■ INTRODUCTION

Allergic rhinitis, even though termed a local disease, it has significant impact on the general wellbeing. It affects social, psychologic, physical, and economic health of a person.

Quality of life (QOL) is affected by:
- Socially unacceptable rhinorrhea
- Affecting quality of sleep (QOS), thereby increasing tiredness and daytime sleepiness
- Reduced academic or work performance
- Aim of treatment of allergic rhinitis
- Restore normal function of upper airway
- Improve QOL
- Improve sleep quality
- Prevent progression of allergic march
- Reduce severity of comorbidities

■ CONTROLLERS IN ALLERGIC RHINITIS

Controller treatment in allergic rhinitis primarily aims in reducing the disturbing symptoms of rhinitis with faster onset of action and thereby improving the QOL and QOS **(Fig. 1)**.

The controller medications include:
- *Antihistamines:*
  - Oral
  - Intranasal
- Anticholinergics
- *Decongestants:*
  - Oral
  - Intranasal
- Mast cell stabilizers

Antihistamines

Antihistamines are the most widely used group of medications in allergic rhinitis. Histamine through its four receptor subtypes (H1, H2, H3, and H4) plays an important role in immunoregulation and acute and chronic

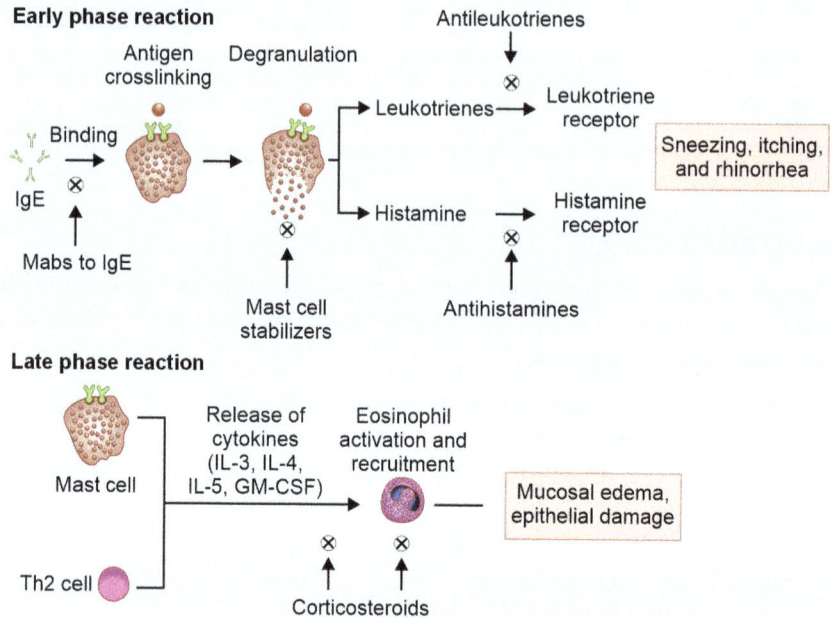

Fig. 1: Site of action of various controller medications. (GM-CSF: granulocyte-macrophage colony-stimulating factor; IgE: immunoglobulin E)

allergic inflammation. H1 and H4 are important in pathogenesis of allergic rhinitis. Histamine released by mast cell degranulation is responsible for early phase symptoms, such as (1) rhinorrhea, (2) itching, (3) sneezing, and (4) vasodilation which cause majority of symptoms in allergic rhinitis.

H1 Antihistamines

Inverse agonists that turn off (combine and stabilize) the H1 receptor and prevent histamine-induced inflammation. As a result, H1 antihistamines prevent and relieve the sneezing, itching, rhinorrhea (early phase response) with small effect on nasal congestion, and conjunctional symptoms (late phase response) **(Box 1)**.

It is broadly divided into:
- First-generation antihistamines
- Second-generation antihistamines
- Third-generation antihistamines

First-generation antihistamine:
- *Example:* Chlorpheniramine, diphenhydramine, and promethazine
- Lipid soluble
- Cross blood–brain barrier

> **BOX 1:** Allergic Rhinitis and its Impact on Asthma (ARIA) guidelines for ideal H1 antihistamines.
>
> *Requirements for oral H1 antihistamines (ARIA guidelines):*
> *Pharmacologic:*
> - Potent, selective H1 block
> - Additive antiallergic activities
> - No CYP3A interaction
> - No disease interaction
> - No food/drug interaction
>
> *Efficacy:*
> - Effective in IAR and PER
> - Effective for all nasal symptoms
> - Effective for eye symptoms
> - *If asthma:*
>   - Improvement of asthma symptoms
>   - Reduction of exacerbations
>   - Improvement of PFT
> - Studies for efficacy in children and elderly
>
> *Side effects:*
> - No sedation
> - No anticholinergic effects
> - No weight gain
> - No cardiac side effect
> - Can use in pregnancy, breastfeeding, young, and elderly
>
> *Pharmacodynamics:*
> - Rapid onset of action
> - Long duration of action
> - No tolerance
>
> (IAR: intermittent allergic rhinitis; PER: persistent allergic rhinitis; PFT: pulmonary function test)

- More central nervous system (CNS) adverse effects
- More cardiotoxicity

Second-generation antihistamine:
- *Example:* Terfenadine, astemizole, loratadine, and cetirizine
- Less lipid soluble
- Block peripheral H1 receptors
- No penetration of blood–brain barrier
- Less CNS side effects
- Cardiotoxic—terfenadine and astemizole

Third-generation antihistamine:
- *Example:* Fexofenadine, bilastine, desloratadine, and rupatadine
- Less cardiotoxicity, CNS side effect
- Faster onset of action
- Longer duration of action

Second and third-generation antihistamines are usually grouped together and are the antihistamine of choice in allergic rhinitis due to its faster onset of action, efficacy both in intermittent, and persistent allergic rhinitis and less side effects.

Adverse Effects of Antihistamines

First-generation antihistamines are sedating drugs because of their lipid solubility and ability to cross blood–brain barrier. They are nonselective and can act on other receptors such as muscarinic receptors causing adverse effects, such as dry mouth, urinary retention, and tachycardia (**Fig. 2**).

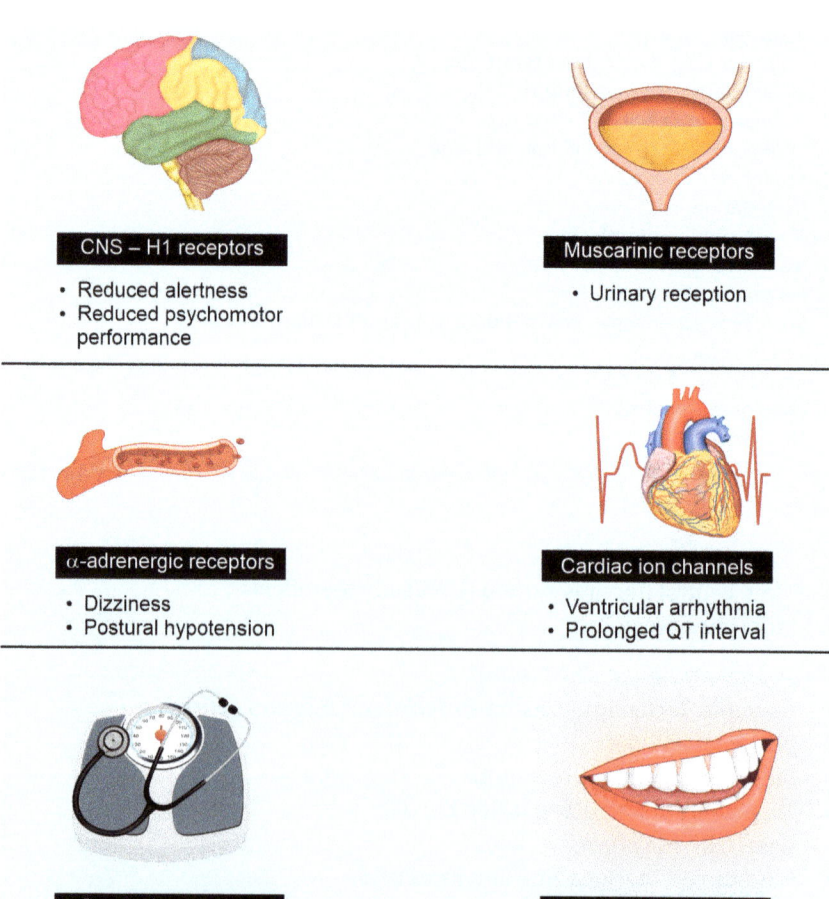

Fig. 2: Adverse effects of H1 antihistamines (primarily first generation). (CNS: central nervous system)

Second-generation antihistamines are less sedating as it is more H1 specific and has less lipid solubility. Cetirizine is the most sedative of second-generation and loratadine and desloratadine are sedative only in high doses **(Table 1)**.

Relative Contraindication
- Patients with QT prolongation
- Pregnancy
- Renal/hepatic dysfunction
- Urinary retention
- High intraocular pressure

Monitoring
- Only in patients requiring prolonged usage, need to monitor for anticholinergic effects.
- ECG—to rule out cardiotoxic effects such as arrhythmia.
- *Toxicity:*
  - Well tolerated
  - No specific antidote
  - Physostigmine—if experiencing delirium

Newer Antihistamines
- *Fexofenadine:*
  - Nonsedative new generation antihistamine
  - Mechanism of action:
    - Selective H1 antagonist
    - Affects inflammatory mediators
  - *Advantages:*
    - Rapid onset of action (1 hour for oral suspension, 1-5 hours for tablet)
    - Long duration of action—OD administration
    - Very less CNS effects
  - *Dosage:*
    - *Adults:* 180 mg OD or 60 mg BD
    - *Pediatric:*
      - Not in children <2 years
      - *2-12 years:* 30 mg BD
      - *If age is >12 years:* 60 mg BD or 180 mg OD
  - *Adverse effects:*
    - Headache
    - Drowsiness and fatigue
    - Dry mouth

TABLE 1: Clinical profile of second-generation H1 antihistamines.

	Cetirizine	Levocetirizine	Fexofenadine	Bilastine	Ebastine	Desloratadine
H1 selectivity	+	++	+	+++	++	++
Peak action	1 hour	0.9 hour	1–3 hours	1.3 hours	2.6–4 hours	3 hours
Duration of action	10 hours	7.9 hours	11–15 hours	14.5 hours	15–19 hours	27 hours
Minimum age	6 months	2 years	2 years	2 years	2 years	1 year
Dosage adjustment in renal disease	Moderate to severe renal dysfunction	Moderate to severe renal dysfunction	Nil	Nil	Careful	Careful
Dosage adjustment in hepatic disease	If associated renal dysfunction	If associated renal dysfunction	Nil	Nil	Careful	Nil
Contraindication	Renal dysfunction	Renal dysfunction	Nil	Nil	Hepatic impairment	Nil
ARIA antihistaminic property	6	6.5	9.5	10	6.5	6.5

(ARIA: Allergic Rhinitis and its Impact on Asthma)

- *Caution:*
  - Dose adjustment in renal disorders
  - Pregnancy (category C)
- *Bilastine:* Newer H1 antihistamine with high affinity for histamine H1 receptors and minimal effects on other mediators.
  - Rapid onset of action: 30 minutes
  - Prolonged duration of action: 16 hours
  - Oral bioavailability: 60%
  - More interaction with fruit juice and drugs
  - *Indication:*
    - Seasonal allergic rhinitis
    - Allergic rhinoconjunctivitis
    - Perennial allergic rhinitis
  - No sedation
  - No dosage adjustment in renal illness
  - No risk of arrhythmia/QT prolongation
- *Ebastine:*
  - Useful for both seasonal and perennial allergic rhinitis
  - Faster onset of action
  - Once daily application
  - Clinical benefit from first day
  - No dosage modification in elderly or those with renal or hepatic involvement

Intranasal Antihistamines

Topical/intranasal antihistamines are used as first-line for relief of symptoms (controller) in allergic rhinitis as per Allergic Rhinitis and its Impact on Asthma (ARIA) guidelines.

Topical H1 antihistamines include:
- Azelastine
- Olopatadine
- Levocabastine

Advantages

- High enough concentration of drug in nasal mucosa for more efficacy
- Effective both in early and late phase allergic reaction
- More effective than oral antihistamines in relief of nasal congestion
- Local antiallergic and anti-inflammatory effects
- Faster onset of action
- Less systematic side effects
- Can be combined with nasal corticosteroids for best results

Disadvantages

- Bitter taste—especially for azelastine
- *Side effects—local:*
  - Dry mouth
  - Swelling of salivary gland
  - Drug rash
  - Headache
- Twice daily application
- Less compliance in some
- Less effective with blocked nose
- Not preferred for long-term treatment in persistent allergic rhinitis

Azelastine Nasal Spray

- *Indication:*
  - Management of seasonal allergic rhinitis in children over 5 years of age and adults
  - Management of symptoms of nonallergic, vasomotor rhinitis ages 12 years and above
- *Dose:*
  - *Children 5-11 years:* One spray each nostril twice a day
  - *12 years and above:* Two sprays each nostril twice a day

Olopatadine Nasal Spray

- *Indication:* Seasonal allergic rhinitis ages 6 years and above
- *Dose:*
  - *Children 6-11 years:* One spray each nostril twice a day
  - *12 years and above:* Two spray each nostril twice a day

Anticholinergics

This group of drugs acts via the parasympathetic pathway. Parasympathetic nervous system stimulation leads to glandular activation which produces watery rhinorrhea. Anticholinergic drugs are effective in blocking parasympathetic-induced release of acetylcholine and block binding of Ach to muscarinic receptors, thereby reducing secretions.

Example: Ipratropium bromide nasal spray

Advantages

- Faster onset of action—within 15 minutes
- Very effective for rhinorrhea by all types of rhinitis
- Can be combined with intranasal corticosteroids

Disadvantages
- Frequent application
- Not effective against other symptoms of allergy such as sneezing and itching

Side Effects
- Transient nasal dryness
- Epistaxis
- Rebound rhinitis (rare)
- *Systemic side effects (rare):*
  - Dry mouth
  - Blurred vision

Preparations Available and Indications
- *0.03% nasal spray:* Management of rhinorrhea associated with seasonal allergic, nonallergic, and vasomotor rhinitis for ages 6 years and above.
- *0.06% nasal spray:*
  - Rhinorrhea of common cold
  - Perennial allergic rhinitis

Dosage
- *Allergic rhinitis:* Two sprays each nostril two or three times a day
- *Seasonal allergic rhinitis:* Two sprays each nostril 0.06% Q6H

Caution
- Narrow angle glaucoma
- Hepatic/renal impairment
- Do not use >3 weeks for allergic rhinitis, 4 weeks for common cold
- Pregnancy (category B)

Contraindication: Hypersensitivity to drug

Mast Cell Stabilizers (Cromoglycates)
Mast cells play an important role in any allergic reaction, both in early phase and late phase.

Mechanism of Action
These are group of drugs which block mast cell degranulation, stabilizing the cell degranulation, stabilizing the cell, and preventing histamine release. They block the immunoglobulin E (IgE)-regulated calcium channels. Without

intracellular calcium, histamine resides cannot fuse to cell membrane and degranulate.

Examples: Cromolyn sodium, nedocromil, antihistamines such as azelastine, olopatadine also has mast cell stabilizing effect.

Preparations

- Nasal Spray
  - Solution
  - Powder for reconstitution

Use

- *Nasal solution:*
  - Prevention of seasonal allergic rhinitis
  - Treatment of symptoms of chronic allergic rhinitis in combination with other drugs
- *Powder:* Prevention of seasonal allergic rhinitis
- *Ocular solution:* For ocular symptoms of allergic rhinitis

Dosage

- One spray each nostril 3-6 times per day (not to exceed 6 times per day)
- Use every day during suspected exposure to allergens (pollen season)

Advantages

- Effective in symptoms such as sneezing, rhinorrhea, and nasal itching
- Can be used as prophylaxis and treatment
- Good safety profile, well tolerated

Disadvantages

- Slow onset of action
- Do not provide immediate relief of symptoms and takes 1-2 weeks.
- Should ideally be used before contact with allergen (prophylaxis)
- Need frequent dosing
- Poor adherence to treatment

Side Effects

- Nasal congestion
- Sneezing, itching, and nasal bleeds
- Rhinoconjunctivitis
- Headache

Caution
- Pregnancy (category B)
- In hepatic dysfunction
- Not effective with nasal polyps

Contraindication: Hypersensitivity to drug

Monitoring: Hepatic/renal function test in patients with hepatic of renal insufficiency

Decongestants

Nasal congestion is the most disturbing symptom of allergic rhinitis. Factors causing nasal congestion include parasympathetic system stimulation and mast cell releasing mediators like histamine, leukotriene, etc. These cause changes in capacitance vessels and increase nasal resistance leading to increased secretions and congestion **(Table 2)**.

Mechanism of Action

Decongestants act by α-adrenergic receptor activation. This leads to vasoconstriction which in turn results in shrinkage of tissue and reduces congestion.

Classification

Based on duration of action:
- *Short-acting local:*
  - *Example:* Phenylephrine
  - Phenylpropanolamine
- *Long-acting oral:*
  - *Example:* Ephedrine
  - Pseudoephedrine

TABLE 2: Efficacy of controller medications in allergic rhinitis.

	Congestion	Nasal itch	Sneezing	Rhinorrhea	Ocular
Oral antihistamines	± (Can worsen)	+++	+++	+++	+
Nasal antihistamines	++	+++	+++	+++	–
Nasal decongestants	++	–	–	+	–
Oral decongestants	++	–	–	+	–
Intranasal anti-cholinergics	+	–	–	+++	–
Intranasal cromolyn	+	+	+	+	–

- *Long-acting topical:*
  - *Example:* Xylometazoline
  - Oxymetazoline

Other decongestant agents are:
- Corticosteroids
- Normal saline
- Hypertonic saline

General Adverse Effects of Decongestants
- *Systemic decongestants:*
  - Nausea and vomiting
  - Insomnia
  - Headache
  - Hypertension
  - Arrhythmia
  - Tachycardia
  - Mydriasis
- *Local decongestants:*
  - Nasal irritation
  - Nasal bleed
  - Rhinitis medicamentosa
  - Atrophy of mucosa—on prolonged use

Phenylephrine: It is the most commonly used decongestant. Primarily $\alpha 1$-adrenergic receptor agonist, thereby causing vasoconstriction and nasal congestion.
- *Onset of action:*
  - *Nasal spray:* 15–30 minutes
  - *Oral solution:* 30 minutes to 1 hour
- *Formulations available:* Nasal spray, oral solution, tablet, topical, and rectal.
- *Uses:*
  - *Intranasal application:* The Food and Drug Administration (FDA) approved for use in nasal congestion related to allergic or nonallergic rhinitis.
  - *Other uses:*
    - Pupil dilation
    - Hemorrhoids
    - Intraocular bleed
  - *As oral decongestant:* FDA has stated ineffective.
- *Adverse effects:* Nausea, vomiting, headache, nervousness, bradycardia, and hypotension can worsen angina and cardiac failure.

- *Dosage:* Nasal drops
  - Approved for >6 months age, one or two drops each nostril every 3 hours
  - >6 years, two or three drops every 3 or 4 hours
- *Disadvantages:*
  - Frequent application of nasal spray, every 3-4 hourly
  - More side effects for oral
  - More drug interactions
- *Caution:*
  - Hepatic, renal impairment
  - Patients with bradycardia and angina
  - Pregnancy (category C)

Pseudoephedrine: It is one of the earliest decongestants.
- *Indication:* Nasal congestion in rhinitis otitis media and sinusitis.
- *Preparations:* Oral, usually available as combination with antihistamine, but more side effects when compared to newer decongestants.

Oxymetazoline and xylometazolines: Alpha agonist with predominant $\alpha 2$-adrenergic activity than $\alpha 1$. Most common over-the-counter (OTC) medication available as nasal spray to treat nasal congestion.
- *Advantage:*
  - Faster onset of action
  - Long duration of action (6-8 hours)
- *Uses:*
  - Nasal congestion of rhinitis
  - Treatment of nose bleed
- *Side effects:*
  - Well tolerated
  - Local side effects, i.e., nasal irritation, nausea, and headache
  - Rare systemic side effects, such as blurred vision, dizziness, headache, hypertension, and nervousness.
  - *Rebound congestion:* Rhinitis medicamentosa, if oxymetazoline used for >4 days and xylometazoline for >7 days continuously.
- *Dosage:*
  - Oxymetazoline:
    - *Adult:* 0.05%; 1-2 drops per nostril 2-3 times a day
    - *Child:* 0.025%
      - 1-6 years of age
      - One or two drops per nostril 2-3 times a day
    - *Baby:* 0.01%
      - If age is <4 weeks, one drop per nostril
      - If age is between 1 month and 1 year, 1-2 drops per nostril

- Xylometazoline:
  - Indicated >6 years of age
  - 6–12 years old, 0.05%, 1–2 drops per nostril
  - If age >12 years of age, 0.1%, 2–3 drops per nostril
- *Caution:*
  - Those with arrhythmia and cardiac disease
  - Pregnancy (category C)

■ SUMMARY

Allergic rhinitis, being a disease with significant impact of QOL, controller treatment plays an important role in faster relief of disturbing symptoms. Proper patient education is essential to spread awareness that controller medication treat only the symptoms, not the cause. Management of allergic rhinitis is complete only with prevention of triggers and definitive treatment.

■ KEY POINTS

- Use of controller medications provides faster relief of symptoms, thereby significantly improving QOL.
- Oral second-generation H1 antihistamines remain first line and most frequently used medication for allergic rhinitis.
- Nasal antihistamines along with nasal corticosteroids remain mainstay of treatment in moderate and severe allergic rhinitis where quicker symptom resolution is needed.
- Intranasal anticholinergic is the drug of choice for treatment of rhinorrhea.
- Intranasal cromolyn is the preferred preventive medication for seasonal allergic rhinitis especially in pollen season.
- Decongestants are the most common OTC medication available for rapid relief of nasal congestion, but have to be used judiciously, weighing the risks against benefits.

■ SUGGESTED READING

1. Abdulla B, Latiff A. Pharmacological Management of Allergic Rhinitis: a consensus statement from the Malaysian Society of Allergy and Immunology. J Asthma Allergy. 2022;15:983-1003.
2. Agostoni JW, Kosak Z, Bartlett S. Allergic rhinitis: rapid evidence review. Am Fam Physician. 2023;107(5):466-73.
3. Bjermer L, Westman M, Holmström M, Wickman MC. The complex pathophysiology of allergic rhinitis: scientific rationale for the development of an alternative treatment option. Allergy Asthma Clin Immunol. 2019;15:24.
4. Brożek JL, Bousquet J, Agache I, Agarwal A, Bachert C, Bosnic-Anticevich S, et al. Allergic Rhinitis and its Impact on Asthma (ARIA) guidelines-2016 revision. J Allergy Clin Immunol. 2017;140(4):950-8.

5. Church DS, Church MK. Pharmacology of antihistamines. World Allergy Organ J. 2011;4:S22-7.
6. Denice KC, Monica L. Treatment of allergic rhinitis. Am Fam Physician. 2015;92(11):985-92.
7. Green R, Feldman C. Treating acute rhinitis and exacerbations of chronic rhinitis—A role for topical decongestants. S Afr Fam Pract. 2020;62(1):5053-6.
8. Lai L, Casale TB, Stokes J. Pediatric allergic rhinitis: treatment. Immunol Allergy Clin North Am. 2005;25(2):283-99, vi.
9. Leceta A, García A, Sologuren A, Campo C. Bilastine 10 and 20 mg in paediatric and adult patients: an updated practical approach to treatment decisions. Drugs Context. 2021;10:2021-5-1.
10. Naclerio R. Anticholinergic drugs in nonallergic rhinitis. World Allergy Organ J. 2009;2(8):162-5.
11. Passali D, Cingi C, Staffa P, Passali F, Muluk NB, Bellussi ML. The International Study of the Allergic Rhinitis Survey: outcomes from 4 geographical regions. Asia Pac Allergy. 2018;8(1):e7.
12. Simons FE, Simons KJ. Histamine and H1-antihistamines: celebrating a century of progress. J Allergy Clin Immunol. 2011;128(6):1139-50.e4.
13. Small P, Keith PK, Kim H. Allergic rhinitis. Allergy Asthma Clin Immunol. 2018;14(Suppl 2):51.
14. Wang XY, Lim-Jurado M, Prepageran N, Tantilipikorn P, Wang de Y. Treatment of allergic rhinitis and urticaria: a review of the newest antihistamine drug bilastine. Ther Clin Risk Manag. 2016;12:585-97.

CHAPTER 11

Preventers

Samyugtha

■ INTRODUCTION

There are various treatment options for allergic rhinitis (AR), including pharmacological and nonpharmacological ones. The treatment aims to prevent future attacks and complications as well as eliminate or lessen the current symptoms. Efficacy, patient preference, tolerability, side effects, and cost are taken into consideration while choosing the right medication. The mainstay of treatment for the condition now includes antihistamines (oral and intranasal), intranasal corticosteroids (INCSs) as well as fixed combinations of INCSs and antihistamines. INCSs or fixed combinations of INCSs with antihistamines dare more effective than oral or intranasal antihistamines. Intranasal treatment is preferred because they have faster onset of action than oral treatments.

■ INTRANASAL CORTICOSTEROIDS

Indication

For persistent AR, INCSs are the first-line treatment and most effective monotherapy in reducing inflammation of the nasal mucosa and conjunctiva. INCSs are more effective than oral antihistamines (OAHs) at treating nasal congestion, pruritus, sneezing, and postnasal drip; however, no discernible improvement has been shown with combination of INCS and OAH over INCS monotherapy. When it comes to treating nasal congestion, which frequently does not improve with OAHs, INCSs are very helpful. However, younger children may be more likely to tolerate an OAH, which is an appropriate therapy, due to age and behavioral constraints. The various INCSs **(Table 1)** do not have significant differences in efficacy, are considered safe, and when used appropriately do not have significant systemic adverse effects. INCSs reach maximal effect after several days to weeks and are best used routinely rather than as needed for severe cases. It is recommended to use INCSs regularly rather than only when necessary for severe cases. They attain maximum efficacy after a few days to weeks.

Mechanisms of Action

Glucocorticoids bind to its receptor in the cytoplasm of inflammatory cells. Receptors get activated and allow the entry of glucocorticoids into

TABLE 1: Intranasal corticosteroids (INCSs).

Name	Common brand name and strength	Onset of action	Systemic bioavailability	Usual adult dose/nostril	Lower age limit	Usual pediatric dose/nostril	Pregnancy grade*	Lactation
First-generation INCS (systemic bioavailability: 10–50%)								
Beclomethasone	Beconase AQ (42 μg/spray)	Few days	44%	1/2 sprays twice daily	6 years	• 6–11 years: 1–2 sprays twice daily • >12 years: Two sprays twice daily	C	Compatible
Budesonide	Rhinocort (32 μg/spray)	3–8 hours	34%	1–2 sprays once daily	6 years	• 6–11 years: 1–2 sprays once daily • >12 years: Two sprays once daily	B	Preferred
Flunisolide	Nasalide (25 μg/spray)	Few days	50%	Two sprays 2–3 times daily (maximum two sprays four times daily)	6 years	• 6–14 years: One spray three times daily or two sprays twice daily • >15 years: Two sprays 2–3 times/day (maximum two sprays four times daily)	C	Compatible
Triamcinolone acetonide	Nasacort (55 μg/spray)	8–10 hours	22%	Two sprays once daily	2 years	• 2–6 years: One spray once daily • 6–11 years: 1–2 sprays once daily • >12 years: Two sprays once daily	C	Compatible

Contd...

Contd...

Name	Common brand name and strength	Onset of action	Systemic bioavailability	Usual adult dose/nostril	Lower age limit	Usual pediatric dose/nostril	Pregnancy grade*	Lactation
Second-generation INCS (systemic bioavailability: <2%)								
Ciclesonide	Omnaris (50 μg/spray)	1 hour	<0.1%	Two sprays once daily	2 years	• 2–11 years: 1/2 sprays once daily • >12 years: Two sprays once daily	B	Compatible
Fluticasone furoate	Flonase Sensimist (27.5 μg/spray)	8 hours	<1%	Two sprays once daily	2 years	• 2–11 years: One spray once daily • >12 years: Two sprays once daily	C	Compatible
Fluticasone propionate	Flonase (50 μg/spray)	2–12 hours	<2 %	Two sprays once daily Or One spray twice daily	4 years	• 4–11 years: 1–2 sprays once daily • >12 years: 1–2 sprays once daily	C	Compatible
Mometasone	Nasonex (50 μg/spray)	Within 12 hours	<0.1%	Two sprays once daily	2 years	• 2–11 years: One spray once daily • >12 years: Two sprays once daily	C	Compatible

*Pregnancy grade [United States Food and Drug Administration (US-FDA) risk category]: Category B: No demonstrable risk to fetus in animal studies with no adequate studies in human. Category C: Adverse demonstrable effect to fetus in animal studies with no adequate studies in human.

the cell nucleus where they bind with glucocorticoid response elements on anti-inflammatory genes. The messenger ribonucleic acid (RNA) for anti-inflammatory proteins is transcribed by these activated genes.

Practical Considerations

- Begin treatment with the highest dosage appropriate for the age. The dose can be "stepped down" to the lowest effective dose at intervals of 1 week after symptoms are sufficiently under control.
- Once-daily dosage preparations are practical and can maximize compliance. With the exception of one, flunisolide, which should be taken twice daily, other formulations have a recommended dosage of once daily.
- Severe cases may need daily use on a chronic basis. Patients with mild or episodic symptoms, as needed use may be sufficient.

Instructions to Patients before Intranasal Corticosteroids Initiation (Fig. 1)

Step 1: Remove the mucus crusts in the nose with saline irrigation and use decongestant if needed.

Step 2: Prime the delivery device as recommended by the manufacturer for first use only.

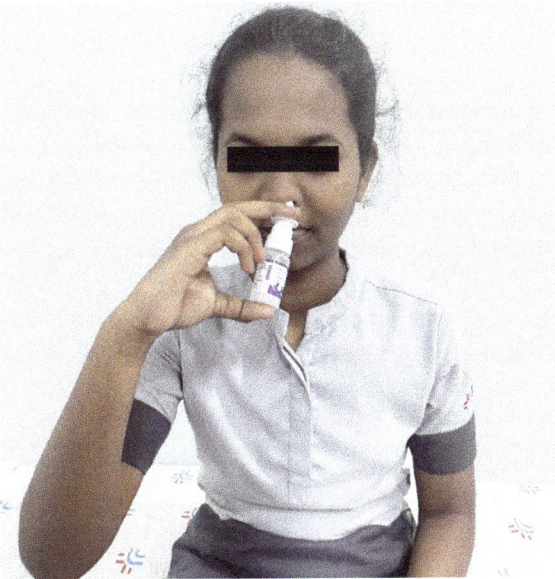

Fig. 1: Demonstration of usage of intranasal corticosteroid (INCS).

Step 3: Positioning—tilt the head pointed forward.

Step 4: Insert the tip of the applicator gently and direct it away from the septum.

Step 5: Aim the applicator tip about 45° from the floor of the nose.

Step 6: Spray and inhale gently.

Adverse Effects

Glucocorticoids generally when used long-term causes stunting in children, decreased bone mineral density, cataract formation, glaucoma, and metabolic effects. Nasal sprays alleviate these long-term complications because of relatively low doses involved and of lower systemic bioavailability. INCSs are grouped into first- and second-generation based on systemic bioavailability. Second-generation INCSs are preferred because of their lower systemic bioavailability (<2%).

Local Effects

- *Local irritation:* Burning and dryness can occur in 2–10% of people. Few people have discomfort from liquid medication running off into their throat. Aqueous preparation causes less irritation compared to alcohol or propylene glycol containing preparations. By employing appropriate administration strategies by tilting head little forward will reduce the discomfort in throat. Dose is gradually tapered to lowest effective dose to minimize these problems.
- *Epistaxis:* When using INCSs, there can be frank epistaxis (uncommon) and scant blood observed in the nasal mucus (common). Blood traces in mucus can be caused by mucosal irritation; this is usually treated by discontinuing treatment on the side where blood-stained mucus is observed for a few days, then commencing therapy again. Repeated spraying may result in frank bleeding due to mechanical trauma and injury to blood vessels. Frank epistaxis is an indication for avoidance of INCSs.
- *Septal perforation:* It is very rare which occurs due to repeated mechanical trauma to nasal septum. Patient must be taught proper administration technique to avoid these complications.

Potential Systemic Effects with Long-term Use

Numerous studies have assessed the possibility of INCSs having systemic absorption, which could have an impact on children's growth and the hypothalamic-pituitary axis (HPA). At approved doses, most have demonstrated negligible or no HPA suppression, particularly when using second-generation INCSs. Studies on first- and second-generation INCSs, however, have indicated a minor impact on growth. Hence, once-daily dosed agents are preferable since they are thought to have less of an influence on growth and HPA, despite lack of supporting evidence.

Drug Interaction

Strong CYP3A4 enzyme inhibitors, such as itraconazole and ritonavir can interact with intranasal fluticasone to effectively enhance the effect of glucocorticoids and cause clinically significant suppression of the adrenal glands. Therefore, individuals on ritonavir, azole antifungals, or other potent CYP3A4 inhibitors should receive treatment with an INCSs other than fluticasone, at the lowest effective dosage.

Monitoring

Growth has to be monitored in children particularly if they are also receiving other glucocorticoid-based treatments, including topical corticosteroids for atopic dermatitis or inhaled corticosteroids for asthma.

SYSTEMIC GLUCOCORTICOIDS

Indication

Oral glucocorticoids taken for brief periods of time (a few days) typically eliminate AR symptoms, and they may be recommended for patients whose symptoms are so severe that they are interfering with their ability to work or sleep.

Mechanism of Action

Corticosteroids decrease the synthesis of cytokines and influence the recruitment, protein synthesis, and survival of inflammatory cells such as eosinophils. They block the expression of adhesion molecules that are involved in remodeling. Systemic corticosteroids decrease the amount of eosinophil mediators (eosinophil-derived neurotoxin, eosinophil cationic protein, and major basic protein) in nasal secretions during the late phase reaction in allergic respiratory diseases (AR).

Adverse Effects

Chronic use may lead to:
- Infections
- Myopathies
- Osteoporosis
- Aseptic necrosis of the femur

- Thinning of the skin
- Hyperglycemia
- Weight gain
- Fluid retention
- Cushingoid appearance
- Neuropsychiatric disorders
- Cataract
- Glaucoma
- Hypertension

Practical Considerations
- Not used routinely in standard treatment for AR
- It can be given to severe and therapy-resistant symptoms, particularly in AR patients who also have nasal polyposis or bronchial asthma.
- Systemic corticosteroids should only be used for brief periods of time—no >5 days—when necessary.

■ LEUKOTRIENE RECEPTOR ANTAGONISTS

Leukotrienes are one of the mediators playing an important role in airway inflammation. Drugs that block their synthesis or their action on receptors helps in reducing airway inflammation.

Mechanism of Action

Leukotrienes are inflammatory mediators produced from arachidonic acid by 5-lipoxygenase in airway inflammatory cells. They are categorized into two groups: those with amino acid moieties and those without. Leukotriene B4 carries hydroxyl moiety only and binds to G protein-coupled BLT receptors to produce chemotaxis response, while cysteinyl leukotrienes (LTC4, LTD4, and LTE4) with amino acid moiety bind to G protein-coupled cysteinyl receptors (CysLT1 and CysLT2) leading to bronchoconstriction, increased vascular permeability, eosinophil recruitment, and chronic inflammation. Montelukast, zafirlukast, and pranlukast are antagonists to cysteinyl leukotriene CysLT1 receptors only. Zileuton is 5-lipoxygenase inhibitor thereby preventing leukotriene synthesis **(Table 2)**.

Indication

Montelukast reduces symptoms of both seasonal and perennial AR. It is mainly used for treatment of chronic asthma and to prevent exercise-induced bronchospasm. Montelukast and oral histamines have similar efficacy but montelukast is inferior to INCSs.

TABLE 2: Leukotriene inhibitors.

Medication	Available preparations	Lowest age limit	Pediatric dose	Adult dose	Adverse effects
Montelukast	• *Granules:* 4 mg/sachet • *Chewable tablet:* 4 mg, 5 mg • *Tablet:* 10 mg	6 months	• *6 months to 5 years:* 4 mg once daily in evening • *6–14 years:* 5 mg once daily in evening	*>15 years and adults:* 10 mg tablet once daily in evening	*Neuropsychiatric events:* Agitation, depression, anxiety, nightmares, insomnia, and suicidal thoughts
Zafirlukast	*Tablets:* 10 and 20 mg	5 years	• *5–11 years:* 10 mg twice/day • *>12 years:* 20 mg twice/day	20 mg twice/day	Headache, dizziness, nausea, flu-like symptoms, abdominal pain, and increased liver enzymes
Pranlukast	• *Capsules:* 112.5 and 225 mg • *Granules:* 50, 70, and 100 mg per packet	2 years	• *2–5 years:* 7–10 mg/kg/day of granules in two divided doses. • *6–11 years:* 7–10 mg/kg/day of granules in two divided doses (maximum 225 mg twice/day) • *>12 years:* 225 mg twice/day	225 mg twice/day	Abdominal pain, diarrhea, and increased liver enzymes
Zileuton	*Immediate and extended-release tablet:* 600 mg	12 years	• *>12 years:* Immediate release—600 mg 4 times/day • *Extended release:* 1,200 mg twice/day	• *Immediate release:* 600 mg 4 times/day • *Extended release:* 1,200 mg twice/day	Headache, dyspepsia, myalgia, sleep disorders, behavioral changes, and liver toxicity

Onset of Action

Montelukast starts to work immediately in reducing leukotriene levels in body, however, it may take up to 2 weeks to reach its full effect.

Safety and Adverse Effects

There is growing concern regarding montelukast's risk/benefit ratio. Montelukast has been linked to neuropsychiatric side effects, including insomnia, bizarre dreams, depression, anxiety, and rarely suicidal thoughts. For patients with AR with coexisting asthma who cannot tolerate or refuse nasal sprays, use of montelukast is justified.

Drug Interactions

Zafirlukast can increase the effect of warfarin thereby prolonging the prothrombin time by 35%. Hence, prothrombin time has to be monitored and warfarin dose has to be adjusted in patients using both. Zileuton increase the levels of theophylline, hence, dose of theophylline has to be reduced to half.

■ COMBINATION THERAPY

Combination Leukotriene Receptor Antagonist/Antihistamine

Symptoms of AR are mainly due to histamine and leukotrienes. Histamine causes rhinorrhea, nasal itching, sneezing, and less of an effect on nasal congestion. On the other hand, leukotrienes increase nasal airways resistance and vascular permeability thereby causing nasal congestion. Studies have shown that newer antihistamines such as bilastine reduced daytime symptoms, such as rhinorrhea, pruritus, sneezing, and nasal congestion and leukotriene receptor antagonist (LTRA) such as montelukast worked better for night-time symptoms, such as difficulty going to sleep, night-time awakenings, and nasal congestion. Hence combination of both can have an enhancing and complementary effect **(Table 3)**. The patients with perennial AR may benefit more from the combination therapy.

Combination Intranasal Corticosteroids/Decongestant Sprays

Because of the potential for rhinitis medicamentosa, it is best to avoid using decongestant sprays alone for a longer period. Intranasal decongestant when combined with intranasal glucocorticoids does not cause rhinitis medicamentosa and studies have shown better improvement in nasal symptoms. Hence, there is a role of this combination in adult patients who do not respond well to intranasal glucocorticoids monotherapy. Intranasal fluticasone furoate-oxymetazoline combination is available in market **(Table 4)**.

TABLE 3: Combination leukotriene receptor antagonist (LTRA)/antihistamine.

Combinations available	Strength	Lower age limit	Pediatric dose[#]	Adult dose[#]
Montelukast-Levocetirizine	• Syrup: 5 mL (4 mg/2.5 mg) • Tablet (4 mg/2.5 mg) • (10 mg/5 mg)	2 years	• Syrup: 5 mL (4 mg/2.5 mg) once daily • Tablet (4 mg/2.5 mg) once daily	Tablet (10 mg/5 mg) once daily
Montelukast-Fexofenadine	• Syrup: 5 mL (4 mg/30 mg) • Tablet (10 mg/120 mg)	2 years	Syrup: 5 mL (4 mg/30 mg) once daily	Tablet (10 mg/120 mg) once daily
Montelukast-Bilastine*	• Syrup: 5 mL (4 mg/10 mg) • Tablet (10 mg/20 mg)	6 years	Syrup: 5 mL (4 mg/10 mg) once daily	Tablet (10 mg/20 mg) once daily
Montelukast-Desloratadine	Tablet (10 mg/5 mg)	12 years	-	Tablet (10 mg/5 mg) once daily

*Taken before 1 hour or after 2 hours of taking food
[#]Once daily doses are preferentially taken in night time.

TABLE 4: Combination intranasal corticosteroids (INCSs)/decongestant sprays.

Available formulations	Brand name and strength	Lower age limit	Pediatric dose/nostril	Adult dose/nostril
Fluticasone furoate-oxymetazoline	Fluticone-OX (27.5 µg/50 µg)	6 years	One spray once daily	Two sprays once daily

TABLE 5: Combination corticosteroid/antihistamine sprays.

Formulations available	Brand name and strength	Lower age limit	Dose/nostril
Azelastine/fluticasone	Dymista (137 µg/50 µg)	6 years	One spray BD
Olopatadine/mometasone	Ryaltris (665 µg/25 µg)	12 years	Two sprays BD

Combination Corticosteroid/Antihistamine Sprays

Intranasal corticosteroid and antihistamine combinations are used in cases where the monotherapy does not work. Bitter taste and headache are reported by few patients using these combinations **(Table 5)**.

■ SUMMARY

Allergic rhinitis in most cases is a persistent condition that requires therapy for a long period. Management includes allergen avoidance, pharmacotherapy and allergen immunotherapy for severe and refractory cases. Glucocorticoid nasal spray is the most effective monotherapy for allergic rhinitis. Second generation antihistamines are preferred due to their minimal sedative effect and comparable effects with older sedating agents. Antihistamine nasal spray can be added if intranasal glucocorticoid monotherapy is not sufficient to relieve symptoms.

■ KEY POINTS

- INCSs are the most effective monotherapy for maintenance in AR. It has only minimal adverse effects when used according to recommendations.
- INCSs are very effective in relieving the nasal congestion.
- Mometasone furoate, fluticasone furoate, and triamcinolone acetonide can be used in children as young as 2 years old.
- Systemic corticosteroids have very limited role in AR. They are used in severe cases for a short duration.
- LTRAs are as effective as antihistamines but less effective than INCSs in AR.
- Combination therapy may be tried in patients not responding to monotherapy and has shown promising effects.

■ SUGGESTED READING

1. Baroody FM, Brown D, Gavanescu L, DeTineo M, Naclerio RM. Oxymetazoline adds to the effectiveness of fluticasone furoate in the treatment of perennial allergic rhinitis. J Allergy Clin Immunol. 2011;127(4):927-34.
2. Berger WE, Meltzer EO. Intranasal spray medications for maintenance therapy of allergic rhinitis. Am J Rhinol Allergy. 2015;29(4):273-82.
3. Borish L. Allergic rhinitis: systemic inflammation and implications for management. J Allergy Clin Immunol. 2003;112(6):1021-31.
4. Bousquet J, Schünemann HJ, Togias A, Bachert C, Erhola M, Hellings PW, et al. Next-generation Allergic Rhinitis and Its Impact on Asthma (ARIA) guidelines for allergic rhinitis based on Grading of Recommendations Assessment, Development and Evaluation (GRADE) and real-world evidence. J Allergy Clin Immunol. 2020;145(1):70-80.
5. Ciprandi G, Tosca MA, Milanese M, Schenone G, Ricca V. Antihistamines added to an antileukotriene in treating seasonal allergic rhinitis: histamine and leukotriene antagonism. Eur Ann Allergy Clin Immunol. 2004;36(2):67-70.
6. Cohen B. Allergic rhinitis. Pediatr Rev. 2023;44(10):537-50.
7. Derendorf H, Meltzer EO. Molecular and clinical pharmacology of intranasal corticosteroids: clinical and therapeutic implications. Allergy. 2008;63(10):1292-300.
8. Dykewicz MS, Wallace DV, Amrol DJ, Baroody FM, Bernstein JA, Craig TJ, et al. Rhinitis 2020: a practice parameter update. J Allergy Clin Immunol. 2020;146(4):721-67.

9. Foisy MM, Yakiwchuk EM, Chiu I, Singh AE. Adrenal suppression and Cushing's syndrome secondary to an interaction between ritonavir and fluticasone: a review of the literature. HIV Med. 2008;9(6):389-96.
10. Gupta R, Fonacier LS. Adverse effects of nonsystemic steroids (inhaled, intranasal, and cutaneous): a review of the literature and suggested monitoring tool. Curr Allergy Asthma Rep. 2016;16(6):44.
11. Hoover RM, Erramouspe J, Bell EA, Cleveland KW. Effect of inhaled corticosteroids on long-term growth in pediatric patients with asthma and allergic rhinitis. Ann Pharmacother. 2013;47(9):1175-81.
12. Valenzuela CV, Liu JC, Vila PM, Simon L, Doering M, Lieu JE. Intranasal corticosteroids do not lead to ocular changes: a systematic review and meta-analysis. Laryngoscope. 2019;129(1):6-12.
13. Wilson AM, O'Byrne PM, Parameswaran K. Leukotriene receptor antagonists for allergic rhinitis: a systematic review and meta-analysis. Am J Med. 2004;116(5):338-44.

Disease Modifiers

R Prasanna

Disease modifiers in allergic rhinitis (AR) include allergen immunotherapy (AIT) and Biologicals. Both will be considered separately in this chapter.

ALLERGEN IMMUNOTHERAPY

■ INTRODUCTION

Allergen immunotherapy (AIT) has been widely used as a desensitizing therapy for immunoglobulin E (IgE)-mediated allergic conditions, such as allergic rhinitis (AR), asthma, and venom anaphylaxis, with some recent evidence in food allergy and atopic dermatitis. It is giving particular allergens to patients repeatedly in an effort to increase tolerance. This improves quality of life by minimizing the need for medicine and relieving clinical symptoms. AIT is generally combined with conventional pharmacotherapy and allergen avoidance strategies.

Allergen immunotherapy is being considered as a disease-modifying treatment with additional preventive effects. The significance of AIT is especially evident in children who have moderate-to-severe AR and do not achieve symptom control despite taking adequate medication. AIT led to a significant decrease in AR symptoms and decreased reliance on medication. Moreover, research suggests a decreased likelihood of acquiring new asthma, in addition to a positive effect on asthma symptoms and drug usage, between 2 and 5 years after receiving either subcutaneous immunotherapy (SCIT) or sublingual immunotherapy (SLIT). These preventive effects are especially noted in children with AR and with pollen allergy.

■ INDICATIONS FOR ALLERGEN IMMUNOTHERAPY
- Features suggestive of AR, with or without conjunctivitis
- IgE sensitization as confirmed by positive skin prick test (SPT) and/or serum-specific IgE to clinically relevant allergens
- Moderate-to-severe symptoms impacting daily activities/sleep despite regular medications and avoidance strategies
- Consideration may be given in less severe AR with pollen allergy to prevent asthma progression.

CONTRAINDICATIONS FOR ALLERGEN IMMUNOTHERAPY

Absolute contraindications are as follows:
- Severe asthma
- Carcinoma under treatment
- Ongoing autoimmune disease
- Insufficient compliance

Relative contraindications are as follows:
- Poorly controlled asthma
- Immunodeficiency
- Serious systemic reactions to therapy in the past
- Severe psychiatric disorders
- Beta-blocker therapy (local or systemic)
- Pregnancy

ROUTE OF ADMINISTRATION

Treatment of respiratory allergic disorders that can improve allergy symptoms by making the immune system adapt to the allergen and reducing the need for medications is referred to as specific immunotherapy (SIT). SIT can be administered through subcutaneous route (SCIT) or sublingual route (SLIT).

Subcutaneous Immunotherapy

It involves the administration of increasing doses by injecting the allergen for 8-12 weeks to reach a maintenance dose followed by injections at monthly intervals for 3-5 years. Maximally tolerated dose (MTD), the dose that results in an undesirable allergic reaction, is sometimes identified and the maintenance dose is given at one or two doses lower than the MTD. It involves giving a conventional schedule (1-3 injections/week for several months during the buildup phase followed by a maintenance phase every 2-4 weeks for an extended period of 3-5 years), rush immunotherapy (where the maintenance phase is usually achieved in days), ultra-rush immunotherapy (maintenance dose achieved in hours), cluster immunotherapy (where allergy shots are administered 1 or 2 days in a week in clusters to achieve maintenance dose) **(Table 1)**.

Sublingual Immunotherapy

It is available in the form of tablets and drops and the main mode of administration is SLIT swallow and SLIT spit as the name implies. The ideal dose for the most optimum response is still under study. The annual cumulative dose is more important for which studies have adopted different dosing schedules. The main advantage of SLIT is the patient can take it at home and need not visit a hospital, unlike SCIT **(Table 2)**.

TABLE 1: Effective dosing for subcutaneous immunotherapy (SCIT).

Allergen	Effective dose	Probable effective dose range of major allergen
Cat dander	1,000–4,000 BAU	15–17.3 µg Fel d 1
Dog	15 µg Can f 1	15 µg Can f 1
Bermuda	300–1,500 BAU	NA
Short ragweed	1,000–4,000 AU	6–12 µg Amb a 1
Birch	3.28–12 µg of Bet v1	3.28–12 µg of Bet v1
Standardized grass	1,000–4,000 BAU	20 µg of Phl p 5 /15 µg of Doc q 5 and Lol p 5
Nonstandardized extracts: Pollen	0.5 mL of 1:100–1:200 weight/volume	NA
Nonstandardized extracts: Mold/fungi and cockroach	Highest tolerated dose	NA
Dust mite: *Dermatophagoides farinae* and *Dermatophagoides pteronyssinus*	500–2,000 AU	7–10 µg of Der p 1 or Der f 1

Source: Adapted from Lao-Araya M, Sompornrattanaphan M, Kanjanawasee D, Tantilipikorn P; the Allergy Asthma and Immunology Association of Thailand (AAIAT) interesting group on immunotherapy. Allergen immunotherapy for respiratory allergies in clinical practice: A comprehensive review. Asian Pac J Allergy Immunol. 2022;40(4):283-94.

IMMUNOTHERAPY FOR PATIENTS WHO ARE ALLERGIC TO HOUSE DUST MITE

House dust mite (HDM) allergens consist of the excrement produced by the species *Dermatophagoides pteronyssinus* (Dp), *Dermatophagoides farinae* (Df), *Blomia tropicalis*, and *Euroglyphus maynei*. Enhanced comprehension of the allergenic properties of proteins has provided vital knowledge for accurate diagnoses and targeted immunotherapeutic strategies to address HDM allergies. Commercially available HDM AIT products can be given via subcutaneous (SCIT) or sublingual (SLIT) routes, with the latter available in drop or tablet forms. Also routes like intralymphatic or epicutaneous are being practiced but not been studied in pediatric populations. SCIT, which utilizes allergen extracts, is recommended for treating perennial HDM AR in children, showing short-term benefits mainly derived from adult studies. Long-term effectiveness needs further investigation. HDM SLIT tablets are recommended for AR treatment in adolescents and adults. HDM AIT can be used either as a single allergen species or a mixture of well analyzed homologous allergens from the same biological family. It is not recommended to use mixtures from unrelated biological families. At present, it is advised to begin HDM AIT at the age of 5 years. There is a lack of research on

TABLE 2: Comparison between SCIT and SLIT.

Characteristics	SCIT	SLIT
Adherence to treatment	Many studies have shown 50% default	Better than SCIT, around 80%
Dosage	Lower than SLIT	3–375 times higher dosage used
Home administration	Never	Always
Route	Subcutaneous	Sublingual
Discomfort	Yes	Rare
Safety	Good safety when used carefully	Better safety profile than SCIT
Cost	Direct cost of antigens is lower, and indirect costs higher	Direct cost of antigens is higher, and indirect costs lower
Patient acceptance	Lower than SLIT	Higher than SCIT
Efficacy: Clinical improvement	Good effect	Good effect but may be slightly less than SCIT. More data is needed and dosage standardized
Efficacy: Prevention of sensitizations	Proved	Data shows that SLIT can prevent new sensitizations
Efficacy: Long-lasting efficacy after discontinuation	Proved	One study has shown an effect lasting after stopping SLIT for 5 years. More studies needed
Efficacy: Switching back to Th1 from Th2	Proved	Recent studies have suggested. More studies are needed
Deaths	Reported in <40 cases in the last nearly 100 years and millions of patients	Never

(SCIT: subcutaneous immunotherapy; SLIT: sublingual immunotherapy)
Source: Adapted from Gupta N. Comprehensive Textbook of Allergy: Striking the Right Balance, 1st edition. New Delhi: Jaypee Brothers Medical Publishers Pvt Ltd.; 2024.

the long-term effectiveness and potential for preventing asthma in children with AR who are sensitive to HDMs.

IMMUNOTHERAPY FOR POLLEN AND OTHER AEROALLERGENS

Pollen Allergen

In allergic individuals, pollen sensitivity usually starts early in life. The development of sensitization to pollen allergens depends on the local pollen exposure profile. Patients typically experience a more complex sensitivity profile as they age, identifying a higher number of allergen sources. Both the sublingual (SLIT) and subcutaneous (SCIT) immunotherapy methods are supported by available scientific evidence. The most well-established subcutaneous and sublingual vaccinations for grass allergy were compared in a recent study, and the results showed that while both had comparable efficacies, sublingual AIT had a stronger safety record. Treatment is guided by selection algorithms based on molecular epidemiological research, electronic diaries, and local aerobiology.

Other Allergens

The use of immunotherapy for cat allergies is supported by just a handful of high-quality evidence. However, the advantages of AIT in the treatment of allergies in canines and other animals including horses, rabbits, and rats have not yet been demonstrated by established clinical data. The use of AIT for mold allergies, mainly through SCIT using *Alternaria* extracts, is supported by low-strength evidence. AITs clinical effectiveness for cockroach allergy is currently being studied.

Studies Done in Patients with Allergic Rhinitis and Allergen Immunotherapy

In 1999, Klimek et al. conducted a meta-analysis of 43 randomized controlled trials (RCTs) involving 1,983 patients with allergic rhinoconjunctivitis (AR), demonstrating the efficacy of SCIT in reducing symptoms and medication use. Ross et al. concluded that SCIT is effective in alleviating AR symptoms based on a meta-analysis of 16 prospective studies. Calderon et al. found SCIT for grass pollen effective in improving AR symptoms and reducing medication use in a Cochrane review. Dhami et al. (2017) reviewed 160 studies, confirming the efficacy of AIT, including SCIT, in improving AR symptoms and reducing drug requirements. Lee et al. observed clinical remission with SCIT for HDM allergy in AR patients. Kim et al.'s meta-analysis favored SCIT over SLIT for AR symptoms in HDM-sensitized patients **(Box 1)**.

Duration of Treatment

- In order to attain substantial clinical efficacy, AIT (both SCIT and SLIT) should be given for a period of 3–5 years.
- Typically, clinical improvement is observed within the first year of therapy.
- To assess clinical benefit, treatment adherence, and consider discontinuation if necessary, patients who are undergoing home-based SLIT should be seen every 3–6 months.
- SLIT should be maintained for a minimum of 3 years following the establishment of clinical benefits.

> **BOX 1:** Practical considerations while starting AIT.
>
> *Facilities:*
> - Expertise in diagnosis and differential diagnoses of AR and allergic asthma
> - Training in recognition and management of severe allergic reactions including anaphylaxis
> - Availability of equipment and trained personnel to manage severe allergic reactions
> - Training in administration of specific AIT products
> - Facilities to observe the patient for at least 30 minutes with SCIT injections and initial dose of SLIT
>
> *Assessing patients and deciding on the best approach:*
> - Effective communication with patients and his/her family about the practicalities of AIT, expected benefits, and potential adverse effects
> - Identification of clinical contraindications to AIT
> - Select an AIT product with documented evidence for efficacy and safety, for the patient's specific presentation, wherever possible
>
> *Undertaking AIT:*
> - Start AIT with SLIT for seasonal allergic diseases at least 2 months, and preferably 4 months before the pollen season
> - Preferably start AIT for perennial allergic disease when allergen exposure is lowest and avoidance measures are in place
> - Dose reductions (usually 50%) or split doses for adverse effects, intercurrent illness, or delayed dosing as recommended by summary of products for SCIT
> - Dose interruption with oral lesions and other issues as recommended by summary of products characteristics for SLIT
> - Facilities to regularly follow up patients promoting adherence to therapy and watching for adverse effects
>
> (AIT: allergen immunotherapy; AR: allergic rhinitis; SCIT: subcutaneous immunotherapy; SLIT: sublingual immunotherapy)
> *Source:* Adapted from Roberts G, Pfaar O, Akdis CA, Ansotegui IJ, Durham SR, Gerth van Wijk R, et al. EAACI Guidelines on Allergen Immunotherapy: Allergic rhinoconjunctivitis. Allergy. 2018;73(4):765-98.

- AIT may be extended for an additional 2 or more years after 3 years of treatment, contingent upon the family and patient's informed decision-making, and the treatment's outcomes.

Causes of Treatment Failure

- Incorrect diagnosis
- Inappropriate duration of therapy
- Insufficient dosage
- Inadequate compliance

Safety of Allergen Immunotherapy

Numerous studies have confirmed that both SCIT and SLIT are very safe in children with AR and well-controlled asthma **(Box 2)**.

> **BOX 2:** Risk factors for systemic reaction during allergen immunotherapy (AIT).
> - Active infection
> - Mast cell disease
> - Systemic response to AIT in the past
> - Severe or uncontrolled asthma
> - High level of sensitization
> - Excessive dose during initiation phase
> - Beta-blocker use
> - Incorrect technique
> - Overdose of allergen extract
> - Intense physical exercise
> - Lack of adherence to the manufacturer's recommendation for dose reduction when changing to a new product batch
> - Ongoing allergy symptoms and potential allergen exposure

ADJUVANTS IN ALLERGEN-SPECIFIC IMMUNOTHERAPY

The effectiveness and biosafety of AIT can be significantly improved by combining it with adjuvants. Adjuvants enhance immune responses specific to allergens, particularly for therapies with low immunogenicity, ensuring safety, inducing a stronger and longer-lasting immune response, and enabling the use of lowered doses. As of now, four adjuvant compounds are commonly utilized in conjunction with AIT: (1) Aluminum hydroxide (alum), (2) monophosphoryl lipid A (MPL), (3) microcrystalline tyrosine (MCT), and (4) calcium phosphate (CaP). Moreover, ongoing research is exploring the potential of novel adjuvants, such as nanoparticles, liposomes, and virus-like particles (VLPs).

NOVEL IMMUNOTHERAPY

- *Allergoid:* Protein is chemically modified for use in AIT to induce immune tolerance. Glutaraldehyde or formaldehyde is used as a cross-linking agent and many allergens can be clustered to form a large molecular weight allergen complex which can induce immune tolerance.
- Molecular modification methods such as recombinant wild-type (wild-type allergens), recombinant hypoallergenic (conformational changes in IgE epitopes), and peptide immunotherapy (short-soluble synthetic peptide or fragments of the allergenic protein) are being tried now.

CHALLENGES AND FUTURE PERSPECTIVES IN ALLERGEN IMMUNOTHERAPY

Challenges and future perspectives in allergen immunotherapy include:
- Need for standardization among allergens
- Unavailability of biomarkers to predict immunotherapy response

CHAPTER 12: Disease Modifiers

- Need guidelines for prescribing immunotherapy in polysensitized patients
- Require more consensus in dosing and schedules especially in children
- Identify newer AIT treatment strategies with better safety profile and efficacy **(Flowchart 1)**

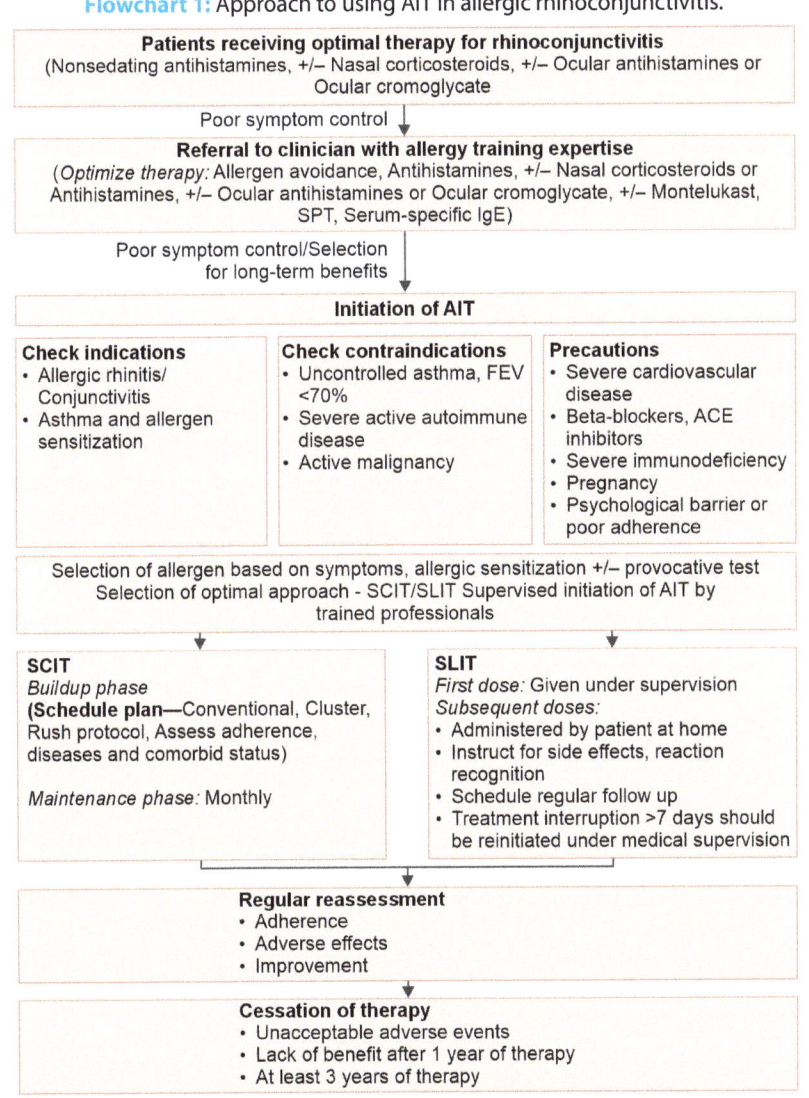

Flowchart 1: Approach to using AIT in allergic rhinoconjunctivitis.

(ACE: angiotensin-converting enzyme; AIT: allergen immunotherapy; SCIT: subcutaneous immunotherapy; SLIT: sublingual immunotherapy; SPT: skin prick test)

Source: Adapted from Roberts G, Pfaar O, Akdis CA, Ansotegui IJ, Durham SR, Gerth van Wijk R, et al. EAACI Guidelines on Allergen Immunotherapy: Allergic rhinoconjunctivitis. Allergy. 2018;73(4):765-98.

BIOLOGICALS

■ INTRODUCTION

Biologicals, large and complex molecules derived from living organisms, are synthesized through genetic engineering processes for targeted actions. These substances interact with specific molecules, cells, or receptors involved in the allergic cascade, disrupting the process at various stages. They exert an immunomodulatory effect by inhibiting the action of proinflammatory cytokines or IgE. Depending on the biological agent's characteristics and the type of allergy, they can be administered via subcutaneous, inhalational, or intravenous routes. Biologicals are typically prescribed for severe allergic reactions that have not responded to conventional treatments. Among them, only omalizumab is approved for use in children under the age of 12 years.

■ MECHANISM OF ACTION (FLOWCHART 2)

Omalizumab, an anti-IgE monoclonal antibody, binds to high-affinity IgE Fc receptors in interstitial region and blood, thereby inhibiting inflammatory cascade. This results in a decrease in the concentration of free IgE in serum, which in turn reduces the binding of circulating IgE to basophils and mast

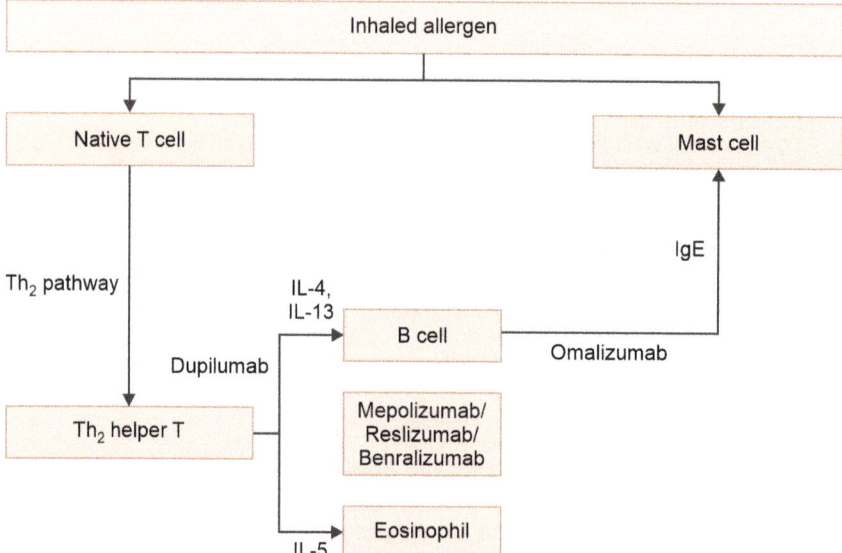

Flowchart 2: Mechanism of action of biologicals.

(IgE: immunoglobulin E; IL-4: interleukin-4)
Source: Shinee T, Sutikno B, Abdullah B. The use of biologics in children with allergic rhinitis and chronic rhinosinusitis: Current updates. Pediatr Investig. 2019;3(3):165-72.

cells. The interleukin-5 (IL-5) pathway is characterized by the activation of Th2 cells, which causes the release of IL-5. This release subsequently enhances IgE levels, eosinophilia, chemotaxis, differentiation, activation, and eosinophil survival. Cytokines that induce Th2 cell differentiation are activated by IL-4/IL-13 pathway inhibitors, which stimulate a type 2 inflammatory response by enhancing the production of eosinophils, basophils, and mast cells, along with the synthesis of IgE. The mechanisms that induce type 2 inflammation, such as mechanical barrier function against the environmental triggers, are facilitated by the cell-mediated cytokine pathway. Additionally, it induces both innate and acquired immunological responses by means of increased cytokine production.

Humanized Anti-IgE Monoclonal Antibody: Omalizumab

Omalizumab works by attaching to free IgE, thereby preventing it from binding to the FcεRI receptor on mast cells and basophils degranulation. Over time, omalizumab downregulates the FcεRI receptors on eosinophils, mast cells, B lymphocytes, and dendritic cells, reducing its expression. This leads to eosinophil apoptosis and prevents antigen presentation by dendritic cells, as well as IgE antibody production by B cells, rendering them anergic.

Dosage

Doses are divided into 150 mg aliquots, with no >150 mg given in a single region, subcutaneously every 4 weeks once for 3-18 months.

Adverse Reactions

Adverse reactions are anaphylaxis and malignancies. Due to the risk of anaphylaxis, it is emphasized that after the first three injections of omalizumab, patients should wait for at least 2 hours. For subsequent injections, patients should wait at least 30 minutes.

Studies Done in Patients with Allergic Rhinitis and Omalizumab

Allergic rhinitis: Tsabouri et al.'s meta-analysis included 11 RCTs and 2,870 patients with seasonal and perennial allergic rhinitis (PAR) and found omalizumab improved daily nasal rescue medication score. Omalizumab was administered subcutaneously every 2-4 weeks at 0.016 mg/kg/IU/mL of IgE, treatment lasted 8-24 weeks (average 16 weeks) and was initiated 4-14 weeks before pollen season. No significant adverse effects were observed.

Birch pollen-induced seasonal allergic rhinitis: Adelroth et al. conducted a study comparing the effectiveness of 300 mg of omalizumab. Patients with IgE levels of 30-150 IU/mL received omalizumab at weeks 0 and 4 (two doses), while those with basal IgE levels >150 IU/mL were given omalizumab at weeks 0, 3, and 6 (three doses). The study noted mildly localized urticaria in three patients. Significant improvements favoring the use of omalizumab were observed in both nasal and ocular symptom severity scores, quality of life, and medication scores.

Seasonal allergic rhinitis induced by Japanese cedar tree pollen: Okubo et al. treated 100 patients with moderate/severe seasonal AR induced by Japanese cedar tree pollen using 150–375 mg of omalizumab in a double-blinded randomized placebo-controlled trial. Post-treatment, there were reductions in nasal, ocular, and medication scores, correlating with lower free IgE levels was observed.

Perennial allergic rhinitis: Chervinsky et al.'s study included 289 patients (12–70 years) with moderate-to-severe PAR lasting 2 years. Omalizumab [at least 0.016 mg/kg/IgE (IU/mL) per 4 weeks] or placebo was administered subcutaneously for 16 weeks. Significant improvements in nasal symptoms, medication use, and quality of life were observed with omalizumab, even in patients unresponsive to other treatments.

Perennial allergic rhinitis and concomitant allergic asthma (SOLAR study): In the "SOLAR" study by Vignola et al., 405 adults and adolescents with moderate-severe PAR and uncontrolled persistent allergic asthma received omalizumab treatment. Over 28 weeks, omalizumab was administered every 4 weeks (0.016 mg/kg/IgE IU/mL). Post-treatment evaluation showed reduced asthma exacerbations, lower symptom scores, and improved quality of life.

Anti-IL-4/IL-13: Dupilumab

Dupilumab binds to IL-4 receptor alpha (IL-4Rα) subunits, blocking IL-4 and IL-13 signal pathways via the common receptor-IL-4Rα. This prevents the end organ response of IL-13 and IL-4 and reduces IgE levels by approximately 40%. Dupilumab has beneficial effects on asthma, atopic dermatitis, and nasal polyps, particularly in eosinophilic asthmatics. Dupilumab has improved the quality of life in asthmatics with chronic rhinosinusitis and nasal polyposis by positively impacting both upper and lower airways.

Dosage
In adults, the dosage is 300 mg/once every 2 weeks; subcutaneous.

Adverse Reactions
Adverse reactions are hypersensitivity reactions, such as urticaria, rash, erythema nodosum, anaphylaxis, and serum disease.

Anti-IL-5 Monoclonal Antibodies: Mepolizumab

Mepolizumab is a monoclonal antibody (IgG1, κ) which targets IL-5, produced by type 2 innate lymphoid cells (ILC2s), Th2 lymphocytes, and mast cells. IL-5 plays a crucial role in eosinophil activation, proliferation, and survival. Mepolizumab has demonstrated significant efficacy and a favorable safety profile.

Dosage

Dosages are 100 mg over 12 years and 40 mg from 6 to 11 years

Adverse Reactions

Adverse reactions are anaphylaxis, angioedema, bronchospasm, hypotension, urticaria, and rash.

Anti-IL-5 Monoclonal Antibodies: Reslizumab

Reslizumab is a monoclonal antibody (IgG4, κ) against IL-5.

Dosage

Dosage is 3 mg/kg (every 4 weeks), intravenous. Infusion (given over 20–50 minutes); >18 years and above.

Adverse Reactions

Adverse reactions are nasopharyngitis, headache, upper airway infections, anaphylaxis, and malignancies.

Anti-IL-5 Monoclonal Antibodies: Benralizumab

Benralizumab is a monoclonal antibody (IgG1, κ) that targets the IL-5 receptor alpha (IL-5Rα) unit, similar to mepolizumab and reslizumab. Additionally, benralizumab binds to natural killer cells, inducing cellular cytotoxicity and apoptosis in eosinophils.

Dosage

Dosage is 30 mg subcutaneous. It is applied every 4 weeks (first three doses) and then applied every 8 weeks.

Adverse Reactions

Adverse reactions are anaphylaxis, angioedema, bronchospasm, hypotension, urticaria, and rash.

Newer Monoclonal Antibodies and Their Targets

Several newer monoclonal antibodies, such as pascolizumab (IL-4), pitrakinra (IL-4Rα), lebrikizumab (IL-13), tralokinumab (IL-13), tezepelumab (thymic stromal lipoprotein), and etokimab (IL-33) are under study for chronic rhinosinusitis with nasal polyps (CRSwNP).

CHALLENGES AND FUTURE PERSPECTIVE OF BIOLOGICALS

Biologicals offer promising treatment options for allergic diseases, but they also present specific challenges.
- Development of cost-effective alternatives or exploring ways to improve affordability
- Better understanding and management of adverse effects
- Understand biomarkers and genetic factors that predict treatment response due to individual variability during treatment
- Efficiency and safety of combining biologicals and other treatments
- Identifying novel therapeutic targets and expanding the range of biologicals available
- Early detection and intervention with biologicals to prevent disease progression
- Longitudinal studies to assess the long-term efficacy and safety of treatment over extended periods.

BIOLOGICAL DRUGS AND AIT: POTENTIAL ALLIES

Evidence indicates combining omalizumab with AIT could benefit respiratory allergies and food desensitization, especially in the build-up phase. Limited clinical trials exist for hymenoptera venom allergy, with single-case reports offering insights. Dupilumab shows promise as adjunctive therapy for respiratory and food allergies, with ongoing trials assessing its efficacy in peanut allergy, multiple food allergies, and as an adjunct to milk AIT. Further research is needed to determine optimal dosing, treatment duration, and patient selection criteria for these therapies.

EFFECT OF OMALIZUMAB ON SPECIFIC IMMUNOTHERAPY IN THE TREATMENT OF ALLERGIC RHINITIS

Omalizumab treatment is utilized in SIT patients with AR for several reasons:
- To minimize the side effects associated with SIT.
- To enable application in high-risk groups.
- To enhance the effectiveness and prolong the SIT treatment.
- To facilitate the tolerance to allergens.

Omalizumab, used alongside SIT, neutralizes IgE, reducing mast cell and basophil IgE expression, and mitigating allergic reactions associated with AIT. In studies by Kuehr et al., Kopp et al., and Casale et al., improvements in symptoms and medication scores were observed when omalizumab was added to SIT. Kopp et al. reported increased disease control during the first pollen season, with fewer local reactions in the omalizumab group compared to the placebo group. Casale et al. found lower allergy scores and reduced risk of anaphylaxis in subjects receiving omalizumab alongside AIT.

SUMMARY

Subcutaneous immunotherapy is a modality of a disease-modifying agent that significantly reduces the new allergen sensitization, however, systemic responses can happen in some children. SLIT has a lot of advantages and is now an important modality in AIT especially in children. Continuous research is being conducted especially AIT use in AR and its progression to asthma. Biologicals on the other hand targeting specific cytokines, receptors, or immune cells have been useful in modifying the course of allergy disease. However, only omalizumab has been well studied, especially in children with AR. Also, safety considerations in their use and careful patient selection are essential to mitigate potential risks.

KEY POINTS

- Allergen immunotherapy is safe, even in children.
- Allergen immunotherapy for HDM is used widely with good results.
- AIT can prevent the march from AR to asthma, especially in pollen allergy.
- Patient selection is key in both AIT and biologicals.
- Omalizumab is a well-studied biological and is useful in AR.

SUGGESTED READING

1. Alvaro-Lozano M, Akdis CA, Akdis M, Alviani C, Angier E, Arasi S, et al. EAACI Allergen Immunotherapy User's Guide. Pediatr Allergy Immunol. 2020;31 Suppl 25(Suppl 25):1-101.
2. Bayar Muluk N, Cingi C. Biologics in allergic rhinitis. Eur Rev Med Pharmacol Sci. 2023;27(5 Suppl):43-52.
3. Carlucci P, Spataro F, Daddato MF, Paoletti G, Di Bona D. Biologic drugs and allergen immunotherapy: potential allies. Explor Asthma Allergy. 2023;1:126-41.
4. Gupta N. Comprehensive Textbook of Allergy: Striking the Right Balance, 1st edition. New Delhi: Jaypee Brothers Medical Publishers Pvt Ltd.; 2024.
5. Halken S, Larenas-Linnemann D, Roberts G, Calderón MA, Angier E, Pfaar O, et al. EAACI guidelines on allergen immunotherapy: Prevention of allergy. Pediatr Allergy Immunol. 2017;28(8):728-45.
6. Lao-Araya M, Sompornrattanaphan M, Kanjanawasee D, Tantilipikorn P; the Allergy Asthma and Immunology Association of Thailand (AAIAT) interesting

group on immunotherapy. Allergen immunotherapy for respiratory allergies in clinical practice: A comprehensive review. Asian Pac J Allergy Immunol. 2022;40(4):283-94.
7. Roberts G, Pfaar O, Akdis CA, Ansotegui IJ, Durham SR, Gerth van Wijk R, et al. EAACI Guidelines on Allergen Immunotherapy: Allergic rhinoconjunctivitis. Allergy. 2018;73(4):765-98.
8. Shinee T, Sutikno B, Abdullah B. The use of biologics in children with allergic rhinitis and chronic rhinosinusitis: Current updates. Pediatr Investig. 2019; 3(3):165-72.

CHAPTER 13

Surgical Intervention in Allergic Rhinitis

Deepak Kumar

■ INTRODUCTION

Allergic rhinitis (AR) is a chronic inflammatory condition of nose and nasal mucosa. Over the years, the incidence of AR is on the rising trend, with up to 24% of the general population suffering from AR, including approximately 30% of the adult population and 40% of children. The hallmark symptoms of AR include sneezing, nasal obstruction, nasal itching, and sneezing. It is sometimes associated with conditions, such as asthma, otitis media, atopic diseases, and various forms of rhinosinusitis.

■ PATHOPHYSIOLOGY

In patients suffering from AR, when the sensitized allergen enters through nose, it leads to influx of inflammatory mediators, which in turn results in mucosal edema, autonomic neural stimulation, and increased mucosal secretions. The inferior turbinates help in modulating airflow resistance through vasodilatation and congestion.

The allergen interaction with nasal mucosa is mediated by dendritic cells (antigen presenting cells), which in turn leads to stimulation of CD4+ T cells via major histocompatibility complex (MHC) class II. Thus, the T cells differentiate to T helper cells type 2 (TH2) which produces immunoglobulin E (IgE) in atopic patients through B cells and proliferation of eosinophils, mast cells, and basophils. This IgE then binds to the FcεRI of mast cells and causes activation of basophils **(Fig. 1)**.

The mainstay of treatment includes allergen identification either by skin prick test or serum-specific IgE followed by strict allergen avoidance. The pharmacological treatments include nasal saline wash, nasal corticosteroids, and antihistamines. The persistent cases are benefited by immunotherapy which acts through desensitization for specific allergen. In refractory cases, where the medical therapy and immunotherapy fails, the surgical intervention can be considered for symptomatic relief. Nasal obstruction is always the most common symptom in the refractory AR, thus the surgery reduces the obstruction and improves the quality of life. The surgery will only reduce the fixed obstruction but it will not reduce the inflammation, for which medical management shall be given.

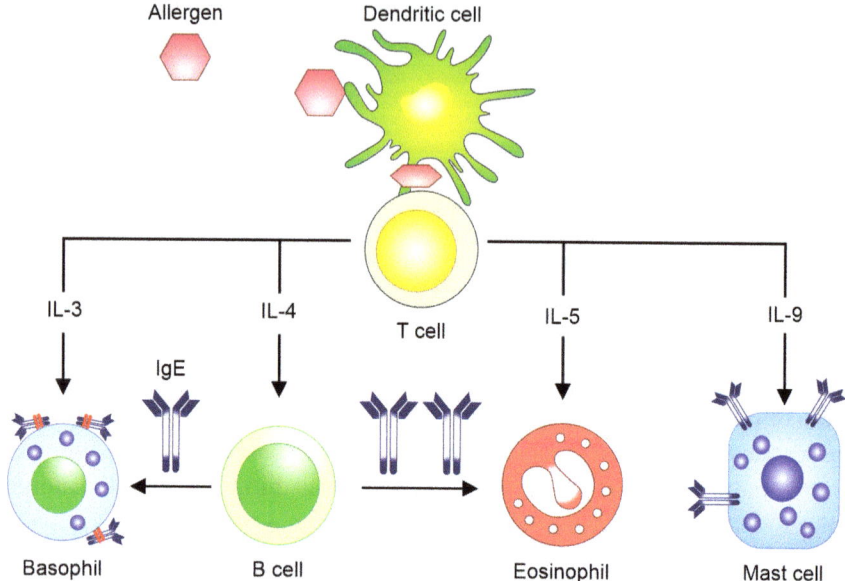

Fig. 1: Allergen-induced sensitization and inflammation. (IgE: immunoglobulin E; IL-3: interleukin-3)
Source: Min YG. The pathophysiology, diagnosis and treatment of allergic rhinitis. Allergy Asthma Immunol Res. 2010;2(2):65-76.

INDICATIONS FOR SURGERY

- Refractory/severe AR
- Failed after conventional medical management
- Nasal obstruction due to structural abnormalities
- Immunotherapy is not indicated/contraindicated.
- Failure of immunotherapy
- Nasal polyps
- Chronic rhinosinusitis

There are many surgical options, such as septoplasty, inferior turbinate reduction (ITR), neurectomy, selective nasal tissue reduction, and endoscopic sinus surgery. Even though the endoscopic surgery has come up in recent years but still the ITR is the most common and most preferred surgery in the refractory cases of AR. The main aim of the surgery of the inferior turbinates is to do debulking of the inflamed tissue or inducing scar formation which will reduce the allergen deposition and its subsequent effects.

COMMON SURGICAL PROCEDURES IN ALLERGIC RHINITIS

- Inferior turbinate reduction
- Lateralization outfracture of inferior turbinate

- Laser vaporization of inferior turbinates
- Submucosal resection
- Radiofrequency ablation and coablation
- Septoplasty
- Endoscopic sinus surgery
- Vidian neurectomy

Inferior Turbinate Reduction in Allergic Rhinitis

The procedure ITR is one of the simplest procedures done for the surgical treatment of nasal blockage. It can be total or radical turbinectomy, though total turbinectomy is now obsolete. The inferior turbinectomy reduces the size of the turbinate which leads to reduction in the net mucosal surface which in turn reduces the allergen contact points and also will increase the room. After surgical removal destroys the vasculature and glandular structure while the upcoming regrowth heals through fibrosis. It will decrease the obstruction and improve the quality of life. There are various techniques which may be used to reduce the size of inferior turbinates such as classic lateral outfracture techniques, submucosal resection, radiofrequency ablation, coblation, and laser reduction.

Lateralization Outfracture of the Inferior Turbinate

In 1904, Killian was first to describe the surgery. The procedure targets the anterior and inferior portion of the inferior turbinates because it is the most resistant part of the airway. The method is displacement of the inferior turbinate in a lateral, then superior, and then inferior fashion until a crunching sound is heard. The benefit of the procedure is that it is simple technique with very few chance of developing atrophic rhinitis whereas it is more in the inferior turbinectomy **(Fig. 2)**.

Laser Vaporization of Inferior Turbinates

Laser therapy is used to ablate the vascular channels of the turbinates which induces fibrosis and reduces the bulk of the turbinates. Some studies suggest complete vaporization of the turbinates but it is not widely accepted. The conventional practice of vaporization is the laser application in a linear fashion, anterior-to-posterior striping, or along only a portion of the turbinate. The laser systems which can be used for the vaporization of turbinates are carbon dioxide (CO_2), diode, neodymium-doped yttrium aluminum garnet (Nd:YAG), potassium titanyl phosphate (KTP), argonian, and holmium:yttrium aluminum garnet (Ho:YAG) lasers. The laser therapy gives adequate response in AR with symptomatic improvement to the tune of 50–100%. The complications associated with the procedure are very minimal.

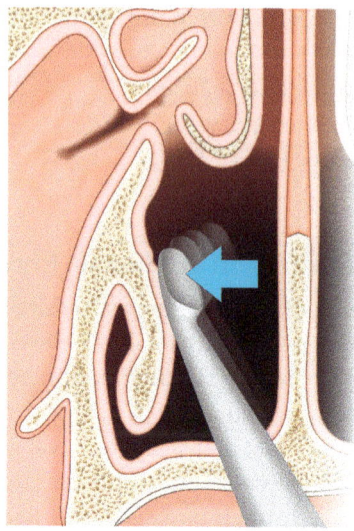

Fig. 2: Outfracture lateralization of the right inferior turbinate.
Source: Chhabra N, Houser SM. The surgical management of allergic rhinitis. Otolaryngol Clin North Am. 2011;44(3):779-95, xi.

It includes crusting, synechiae formation, and sometime bony exposure to nasal structure. But, the cost of machine and procedure lead to nonavailability at most of the centers.

Submucosal Resection

The main goal of the procedure is to reduce in size of the bulky inflammatory tissue with maximal preservation of the mucosa for maintaining the ciliary function.

The submucosa resection involves an incision and a mucosal flap elevation on the medial side of the inferior turbinate, followed by forceps resection of the bone. The lateral mucosa overlying the inferior meatus was sometime removed as well, whereas the conserved mucosa on the medial aspect was then redraped over the resected bone **(Fig. 3)**.

Radiofrequency Ablation and Coablation

Radiofrequency ablation technique in which the probe is inserted in the inferior turbinates and low frequency ionic energy is delivered. This postoperatively results in contracture and fibrosis but the ciliary function and epithelium is preserved. The procedure produces significant symptomatic improvement with less or no side effects as compared to other form of turbinoplasty.

CHAPTER 13: Surgical Intervention in Allergic Rhinitis

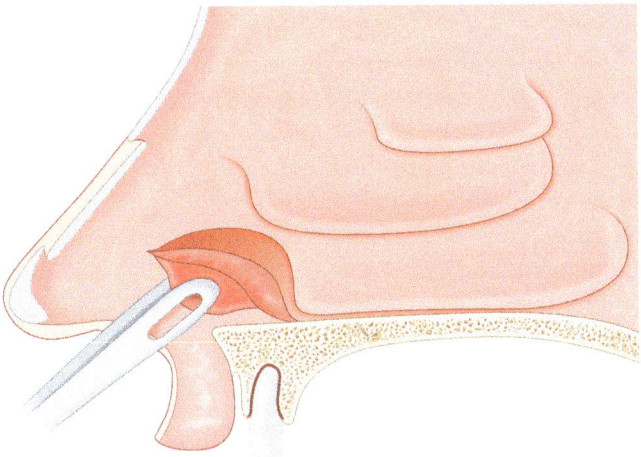

Fig. 3: Submucous resection of the lower turbinate.
Source: Chhabra N, Houser SM. The surgical management of allergic rhinitis. Otolaryngol Clin North Am. 2011;44(3):779-95, xi.

The coblation is under the umbrella term of radiofrequency ablation which exploits molecular ionization to achieve low temperature and it focuses on disintegration of the tissue. This technique is preferred in pediatric population because of less complication like pain.

Septoplasty

No doubt the inferior turbinates show significant changes in AR but the anatomical changes of the nasal septum affects the laminar flow of the air flow in the nasal cavity. Some researchers have found that septoplasty is not a good option for AR but many studies concluded that the septoplasty is not indicated alone and it has to be combined with turbinoplasty or endoscopic sinus surgery, especially when obvious anatomic deformity is present.

Endoscopic Sinus Surgery

The endoscopic surgery is most common procedure in nasal obstruction due to chronic rhinosinusitis, polyp, and allergic fungal sinusitis but it is not a good modality for AR. The endoscopy in chronic sinusitis helps to maximize the patency of the airways and alleviates the effects of edematous ostia. The endoscopic removal of the polyp which occludes the osteomeatal complex or nasal fossa. It is very much helpful in the debridement of thick inspissated mucus secretion in allergic fungal sinusitis. The endoscopic surgery may be combined with turbinoplasty in refractory or severe cases of AR.

Vidian Neurectomy

In 1961, Golding-Wood described the procedure vidian neurectomy. It is the transection of parasympathetic reflexes. The surgery is now of historical importance only because of adverse outcomes it is not of much importance. The vidian nerve is formed by the union of superficial and greater petrosal nerve and the pericarotid plexus before joining the sphenopalatine ganglion. The procedure reduces hyperreactivity of the nasal reflex, effectively reducing sneezing and nasal hypersecretion. The side effects include keratoconjunctivitis sicca, eye movement disorders, abducens paralysis of eye.

■ SUMMARY

The AR is the condition and it is mainly treated by medical management and allergen avoidance. In refractory cases of AR, surgery is indicated where the nasal obstruction is so severe that the symptom compromises the quality of life. The inferior turbinates hypertrophy is the culprit for nasal obstruction of the airways in AR. There are many procedures to reduce the airways because no modality is gold standard. It totally depends on the surgeon and the condition of the patient decides the approach of surgery.

■ KEY POINTS

- Allergic rhinitis is a widespread condition with common symptoms of nasal obstruction, sneezing, nasal itching.
- In cases of allergic rhinitis refractory to medical treatment, surgical intervention maybe necessary.
- In surgical management the inferior turbinate reduction/debulking is the main goal of augmenting the airway passage.
- A variety of surgical procedures exist which includes out fracture, sub mucous resection, laser vaporization, radiofrequency ablation, and coablation.
- No single operation has evolved as the gold standard for treatment of nasal obstruction in allergic rhinitis.

■ SUGGESTED READING

1. Aksoy F, Yldrm YS, Veyseller B, Ozturan O, Demirhan H. Midterm outcomes of outfracture of the inferior turbinate. Otolaryngol Head Neck Surg. 2010;143(4):579-84.
2. Bousquet J, Van Cauwenberge P, Khaltaev N; Aria Workshop Group; World Health Organization. Allergic rhinitis and its impact on asthma. J Allergy Clin Immunol. 2001;108(5 Suppl):S147-334.
3. Chang CW, Ries WR. Surgical treatment of the inferior turbinate: new techniques. Curr Opin Otolaryngol Head Neck Surg. 2004;12(1):53-7.

4. Chhabra N, Houser SM. The surgical management of allergic rhinitis. Otolaryngol Clin North Am. 2011;44(3):779-95, xi. (Figures 1 and 2).
5. Fjermedal O, Saunte C, Pedersen S. Septoplasty and/or submucous resection 5 years nasal septum operations. J Laryngol Otol. 1988;102:796-8.
6. Golding-Wood PH. Observation of petrosal and vidian neurectomy in chronic vasomotor rhinitis. J Laryngol Otol. 1961;75:232-47.
7. Houser SM. Surgical treatment for empty nose syndrome. Arch Otolaryngol Head Neck Surg. 2007;133(9):858-63.
8. Passali D, Lauriello M, Anselmi M, Bellussi L. Treatment of hypertrophy of the inferior turbinate: long-term results in 382 patients randomly assigned to therapy. Ann Otol Rhinol Laryngol. 1999;108(6):569-75.
9. Stoksted P, Gutierrez C. The nasal passage following rhinoplastic surgery. J Laryngol Otol. 1983;97:49-54.
10. Wolfson S, Wolfson LR, Kaplan I. CO_2 laser inferior turbinectomy: a new surgical approach. J Clin Laser Med Surg. 1996;13:81-3.
11. Worldwide variation in prevalence of symptoms of asthma, allergic rhinoconjunctivitis, and atopic eczema: ISAAC. The International Study of Asthma and Allergies in Childhood (ISAAC) Steering Committee. Lancet. 1998;351(9111):1225-32.
12. Wright AL, Holberg CJ, Martinez FD, Halonen M, Morgan W, Taussig LM. Epidemiology of physician-diagnosed allergic rhinitis in childhood. Pediatrics. 1994;94(6 Pt 1):895-901.

SECTION 4

Prevention, Alternative Medicine, and the Way Ahead

Section Editor: *Rupali Patil Jain*

- **Preventive Measures**
  Amit Suyal

- **Evidence-based Complementary and Alternative Medicine for Allergic Rhinitis**
  Kashinath G Metri

- **Futuristic View**
  Rupali Patil Jain

CHAPTER 14

Preventive Measures

Amit Suyal

■ INTRODUCTION

Most atopic diseases have their origin traced back to early childhood and hence the interventional strategies also need to trace backward to the origin, i.e., during the period of pregnancy and early infancy to nip it in the bud. This marks the beginning of preventive medicine in the era of allergy.

The prevalence of allergic rhinitis (AR) is about 5% in age group 3 years and progressively goes to 8.5% (6-7 years old) to 14.6% (13-14 years) and a staggering 46% (20-44 years age group), the preventive aspect of allergy plays a more so important role in keeping the allergy process under check.

Preventive aspects of various allergic diseases have more or less similar approach conceptually and since AR forms a part of the spectrum of allergic march phenomenon comprising atopic dermatitis, food allergies, airway allergies (AR + Asthma), the preventive measures mentioned below generally apply to these diseases mentioned above but with special reference to AR.

There are three modes of prevention conventionally, viz.,

1. *Primary prevention:* Primary prevention means stopping the beginning of an allergic disease.
2. *Secondary prevention:* Secondary prevention means halting the progression and exacerbation of allergic disease.
3. *Tertiary prevention:* Tertiary prevention is all about decreasing the disease load in patients who have full blown manifestations of allergic diseases by allergen immunotherapy (AIT) or with the help of medical rehabilitation.

With regards to allergic diseases perse, a fourth mode of prevention suitably called "fourth prevention" is also mentioned which involves preventing relapses of allergic disease once the patient has been completely asymptomatic for a considerable time duration. Among those who benefit most are adolescents who need to be enlightened about no smoking practices and refraining from surroundings which are smoke-filled like discotheques. Pulmonary function needs to be assessed in these individuals on an annual basis and immediate action should be taken even with the onset of mildest respiratory symptoms. Of great importance is the career guidance to choose occupations which refrain from regular contact with potential allergens or irritants in workplace.

All these are graphically depicted in the **Figure 1**

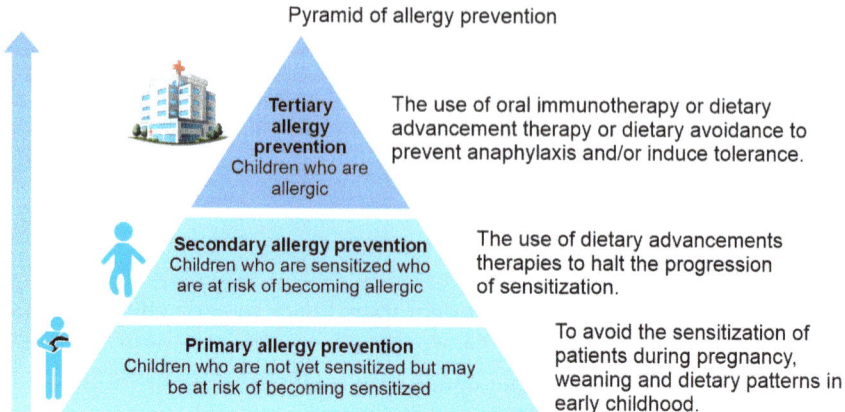

Fig. 1: Three tiers of allergy prevention.

Although the primary mode of prevention is the best mode of prevention for any allergic disease, its feasibility is very challenging in the real-world scenario as it primarily involves the identification of at-risk patients before they start manifesting allergies. Hence, a thorough family history of children born to atopic parents with close sequential monitoring becomes a vital part of identifying the atopic manifestations and intervening early.

■ INTERVENTIONS UNDER PRIMARY PREVENTION
Environmental Factors

- *Microbiota and microbial exposure:* David Strachan in 1989 gave a hygiene hypothesis and now several years later with numerous studies backing it, it has been shown that microbes (both environmental and commensals inhabiting our body) have a crucial role in inducing tolerance by stimulating regulatory T and B cells. The biodiversity hypothesis and many farm studies have showed the protective nature of exposure to cattle, their sheds, and even consuming unprocessed cattle milk from early childhood mainly due to abundance of bacteria and fungi in the rural atmosphere. One study of the named LUKAS done in finnish population has showed that microbiota in nonfarm houses was as beneficial as contemporary farms and had similar allergy protective effect.
- *Pets:* Owning a pet dog(s) and their close interaction with growing children has shown protective effects from allergy to food and house dust mite (HDM) sensitization. The reason behind this protective phenomenon is the increased microbial diversity in homes with dogs exhibiting fourfold more bacterial species compared to homes without dogs. Although a cat's role in allergy protection is slightly controversial, Hesselmar et al. showed that kids exposed to cats in their first year of life were rarely

TABLE 1: Furry animals: characteristics of allergen exposures in residential and nonresidential environments.*

Domestic	Dust	Airborne		
Cats (dander)	++ to +++	+ to ++	?	± to ++†
Dogs (dander)	++ to +++	+ to ++	Yes	± to ++
Pets				
Guinea pig	?	?	?	
Hamsters (dander)	?	?	?	Not known
Rabbits	++ to +++	?		Likely
Mice (urine)	Rare	++	?	Not known
Rats (urine)	Rare	+	?	Not known
Pests				
Mice (urine)	+ to +++	+++		Likely
Rats (urine)	Yes	2		Not known
Laboratories	*In the laboratory*			
Mice (urine)	++	+ to +++	?	Little known
Rats (urine)	++	+ to +++	?	Little known
Farms and stables	*In stable*	*At home*		
Horses	+++	Yes	?	Assumed
Cows	+++	+ to ++	?	Rare

(+: Measurable levels but contribution to sensitization or symptoms is less clear; ++: Levels consistent with sensitization and symptoms; +++: Levels consistently higher than those known to cause sensitization)
*Data were derived from discussions at the workshop and published data.
†Airborne cat allergen has been measured in homes without a cat.

skin prick test (SPT) positive to cat antigen in their teen age. So, in general; common household pets like dogs and cats do impart a protective effect on the humans in close vicinity to them. **Table 1** gives an overview of different pets and their effect on allergies.

- *C-section:* Contact with maternal vaginal flora during birthing has been proven to positively influence the newborn's skin and gut microbiota which in turn stimulates the Th1 pathway and overpowers the Th2 pathway dominant in all fetuses. Studies have shown that babies born through C-sections with or without indication have an increased prevalence of food and airway allergies in childhood.
- *Day care:* Children who attend day care in their childhood days are at decreased risk of sensitization to food/aeroallergens/atopic dermatitis, and asthma development. This can be interpreted as slowing or even halting the allergic march. The same phenomenon is also seen in families with many children and is aptly labeled as sibling effect.

- *Exposure to molds:* Exposure to indoor mold especially in moist homes is a risk factor for respiratory allergies. Getting rid of indoor molds is an important primary prevention for allergic respiratory disorders such as rhinitis and asthma.
- *Exposure to tobacco smoke:* Risk of respiratory allergies in general and asthma, in particular, is increased by at least 25% in the offspring of active and passive smoking parents. Vaping and e-cigarettes also have shown similar adverse effects.
- *House dust mite exposure:* Although HDM sensitization is ubiquitous in most of us and is also a known contributing factor for perennial allergic diseases such as AR and bronchial asthma, the avoidance measures for dust mite alone or in combination have not proven to be of any significant help in preventing the sensitization and allergic manifestations in an individual. Allergen-specific immunotherapy (SIT) which is a secondary and tertiary prevention strategy is the only modality proven to alter the natural course of disease in the case of dust mites.
- *Pollen:* Pollen sensitization is an important trigger of seasonal allergies and affects 10–30% of the global population. Due to global warming, the pollen seasons have increased duration and even trees are producing larger quantities of pollens resulting in more severe symptoms. Humidity and thunderstorms rupture the pollen grains and release microscopic starchy fragments into the atmosphere which have high allergic propensity due to their sheer microscopic size and easy access to deeper respiratory passages. High-efficiency particulate air (HEPA) filters can be of help if used judiciously in seasonal allergies. Pollen immunotherapy is a successful modality in pollen allergy providing long-term relief even after discontinuation.

Climate Change and Air Pollution

Air pollution consists of traffic-related air pollution (TRAP) molecules such as carbon, NO_2, NO, SO_2, CO, and CO_2. Climate change and increasing TRAP directly impact the global load of allergic diseases, hence global programs for combating pollution and climate change could have a beneficial effect in reducing allergy prevalence.

Dietary Intervention and Strategies

- *Prebiotics and probiotics:* Though still not backed by evidence completely, prophylaxis with pre- and probiotics may be beneficial in high-risk kids. Probably this is the reason why the World Allergy Organization (WAO) encourages prebiotic supplementation to all babies who are not breastfed and probiotics in pregnancy and early childhood in those children who are at high risk of developing allergy.

	Beneficial allergy prevention strategies	Research needs
Global environment	• Reduction in traffic-related air pollution	• Impact assessment of air pollution and climate change on allergic diseases
Local environment	• Environment of rich and diverse bacteria species • Cigarette-smoke free environment • Less indoor moisture and molds	• Exact definition of protective microbial composition
Individual behavior	• Dietary supplements in pregnancy might be beneficial • Natural birth might be beneficial • Early introduction of diverse solid food	• Prevention studies based on individual risk assessment with novel biomarkers

Fig. 2: Prevention strategies and research needs to decrease allergic diseases at individual, local, and global level.
Source: Traidl-Hoffmann C, Zuberbier T, Werfel, T. Allergic Diseases – From Basic Mechanisms to Comprehensive Management and Prevention. Switzerland AG: Springer Nature; 2021.

- *Vitamin D:* Evidence is lacking in its role in preventing allergy and hence vitamin D supplementation is not recommended allergic disease prevention.
- *Long-chain polyunsaturated fatty acid (LC PUFA) and fish oil supplements:* LC PUFAs and fish oil capsules consumption in early childhood did not show any benefit in AR and atopic dermatitis risk; however, some benefit was seen in reduced risk of asthma.
- *Breastfeeding:* Although no evidence for allergy and asthma prevention exists as randomized controlled trial (RCT) studies are unethical with regards to breastfeeding. It is highly recommended for the first 4 months of life.

Figure 2 depicts a list of beneficial allergic interventions at the individual, local, and global levels.

As the primary prevention is not from being widely implemented effectively, secondary and tertiary prevention have a considerable role in allergy management.

SECONDARY PREVENTION

Secondary prevention is all about preventing the progression and exacerbation of allergy.

Early and timely intervention with optimal use antiallergic and anti-inflammatory medications forms the crux of secondary prevention and it helps in improving the quality of living in allergic patients.

In sensitized patients, in addition to pharmacotherapy secondary prevention also incorporates allergen avoidance and AIT.

The European Academy of Allergy and Clinical Immunology (EAACI) task force on AIT for allergy prevention endorses AIT in patients having mild AR because it modifies the disease course.

TERTIARY PREVENTION

Tertiary prevention is all about decreasing the disease burden in people with proven disease by AIT and/or medical rehabilitation.

There is moderate-to-high quality evidence regarding the subcutaneous immunotherapy (SCIT) or sublingual immunotherapy (SLIT) in patients with moderate or severe AR with suboptimal control despite pharmacotherapy and evidence says that the benefit lasts even after 2 years post AIT.

Medical Rehabilitation

Medical rehabilitation is employed in the treating chronic diseases and consists of multidisciplinary treatment through a team of healthcare workers.

Although AR perse does not generally need medical rehabilitation, AR is a part of the allergic spectrum which culminates in severe respiratory disability if left unchecked. Almost 65.24% of asthmatics have coexisting AR. The main goal of medical rehabilitation is to ensure a better quality of life and controlling or slowing the progression of disease.

The following are the key components that form part of medical rehabilitation:
- *Patient education:* The goal is to impart correct knowledge of the disorder which in turn, leads to a better awareness and self-care, thus positively influencing the quality of life.
- *Psychological and behavioral interventions:* These interventions look into psychological comorbidities, such as anxiety, depression, and panic attacks in patients with difficult-to-control diseases. It involves improving the emotional state of the patient, boosting self-confidence, and resolving any sleep-related issues. Also, counseling on social and professional problems is being dealt appropriately.
- *Multidisciplinary treatment plan:* This involves a team approach to cater to many issues that may crop up because of AR perse or allergy as a major underlying phenomenon with AR being just a part of the spectrum of allergic diseases. The team incorporates healthcare specialties from different disciplines, specialized nurses, respiratory therapists, psychologists, etc.

ALLERGEN-SPECIFIC PREVENTION

Preventive allergy treatment (PAT) study has evaluated the role of allergen-SIT in delaying asthma onset in kids with proven AR.

The asthma onset was delayed by three times when SIT was administered compared to placebo in children with proven cases of AR.

This narrow spectrum prevention strategy targeted to only sensitized antigens with SIT is more beneficial than blanket approach targeted to influence the immune response to environmental antigens.

ALLERGEN-SPECIFIC IMMUNOPROPHYLAXIS OF ALLERGIC RHINITIS

The evidence of the molecular-spreading process in AR invites for an earlier immunological intervention directed toward preventing its clinical manifestations. Holt's proposal of an "immunoprophylaxis of atopy" can be applied not only at the "primary" prevention level (i.e., to nonsensitized at-risk children), but even at "secondary" allergen-specific immunoprophylaxis (SIP), targeted to children who are healthy clinically but sensitized to grass pollen. The PAT study has proved the disease-modifying potential of AIT when applied early enough. This phenomenon can be easily understood by an example as depicted in **Figure 3**.

Allergen control forms an important basis in the management of AR and as the main objective is to restore the functionality of upper airways and improve the quality of life, it becomes important to enforce allergen control measures apart from imparting pragmatic knowledge to the patient regarding the disease. The control measures can be grouped under three main headings as follows:
1. Environmental measures
2. Individual measures
3. Combined measures

Let us elaborate on each of the above with the available evidences in support of them.

Environmental Measures

- *Air purifier systems [high-efficiency particulate air (HEPA) filter units]:* Numerous studies have shown that the air purifiers do not help in controlling the most common culprit allergen for perennial allergic rhinitis (PAR), i.e., HDM. There was neither a decrease in HDM allergen levels nor was there any improvement in the severity of symptoms and quality of life as a whole. So, in patients with PAR air purifiers do not offer any benefit with regards to quality of life improvement.

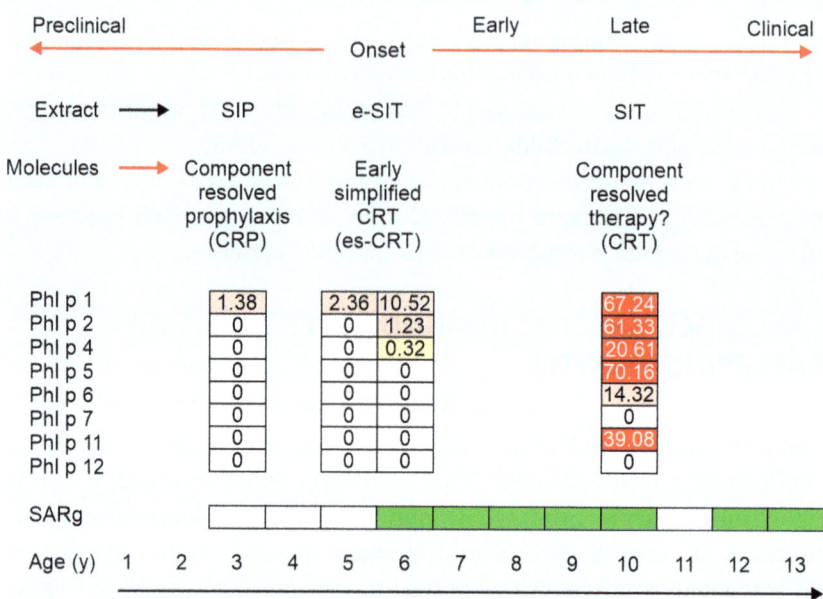

Fig. 3: Molecular spreading of the IgE response to Timothy grass and potential implications for allergen-specific immunologic intervention in a child with seasonal allergic rhinitis to grass pollen (SARg). Molecular spreading of the IgE response to *Phleum pratense* and implications for allergen-specific immunological intervention in one child with hay fever (case from the MAS birth cohort). This child started suffering from hay fever symptoms at the age of 6 years. IgE response against *P. pratense* started 3 years before with a weak, monomolecular sensitization to Phl p 1. This IgE response was stronger and directed also to Phl p 2 and Phl p 4 at disease onset. After disease onset, the IgE response was much stronger and directed also to Phl p 5, Phl p 6, and Phl p 11. In clinical practice, allergen-specific immunotherapy (SIT) would be "normally" prescribed at this advanced stage, after some years of symptoms (age 10 years). An interesting hypothesis is that SIT would be more efficient if started much earlier, ideally "at" disease onset (age 6 years) (early SIT). Moreover, it could be investigated whether an immune intervention at the earliest, preclinical stages (age 3 years) of disease could even better change the natural history of the sensitization and prevent or delay diseases onset [allergen-specific immunoprophylaxis (SIP)]. The use of recombinant allergens would be easier at this stage, as less molecules should be used [component-resolved immune prophylaxis (CRP)]. (IgE: immunoglobulin E; MAS: Multicenter Allergy Study)
Source: Reprinted with the permission of Wolters Kluwer Health License, first published in Matricardi PM. Molecular profile clustering of IgE responses and potential implications for specific immunotherapy. Curr Opin Allergy Clin Immunol. 2013;13(4):438-45.

- *Fresh air ventilator systems (pollen filter units):* These air purifiers equipped with pollen filters have proven to be particularly useful in abating the symptoms in patients with seasonal allergic rhinitis (SAR). There was an improvement in allergy scores and overall quality of life.

- *Temperature and humidity control machine:* This mode of intervention has proven to be successful in PAR children sensitized to HDM. Manuyakorn et al. devised the temperature and humidity control machine as shown in **Figure 4**. The temperature is maintained at 25°C and relative humidity at 55%. After 2 months of continuous usage of the machine, there was a statistically significant improvement in the total nasal symptom score (TNSS) of enrolled children with PAR.

Also, the continuous usage of the machine showed a decrease in the quantitative level of the HDM antigen in the room. Mohan et al. replicated

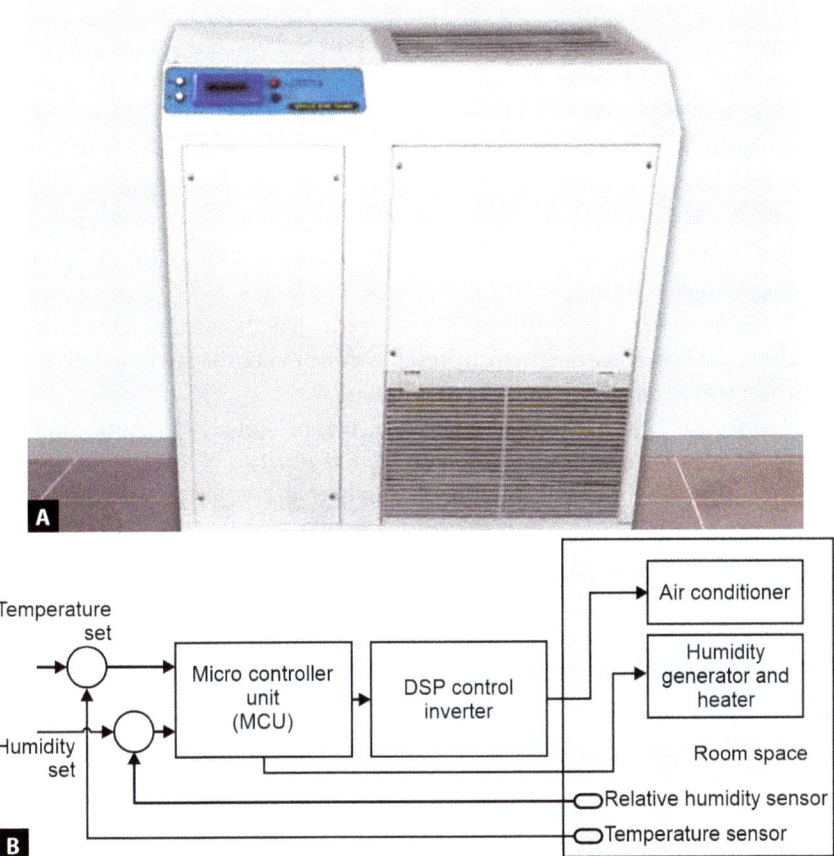

Figs. 4A and B: (A) The newly invented temperature and humidity control machine; (B) The operating system of the machine with air conditioner. (DSP: Digital signal processors)
Source: Manuyakorn W, Padungpak S, Luecha O, Kamchaisatian W, Sasisakulporn C, Vilaiyuk S, et al. Assessing the efficacy of a novel temperature and humidity control machine to minimize house dust mite allergen exposure and clinical symptoms in allergic rhinitis children sensitized to dust mites: a pilot study. Asian Pac J Allergy Immunol. 2015;33(2):129-35.

a similar experiment but only controlled the temperature by using the temperature-controlled laminar airflow system, however, this modality did not show improvement in either symptom reduction or improving sleep quality.
- *Bed covers/mattresses:* Studies done on the role of mite-proof bed covers, showed there was a reduction in the level of HDM antigen, but no improvement was seen in the visual analog scale (VAS) score or daily symptom score of these patients.
- *Probiotics-impregnated bed covers:* Berings et al. in their study showed there was an improvement in overall symptom scores and quality of life in the intervention group that used their probiotic mattresses. These mattresses were manufactured using Purotex® textile treatment which contains five different strains of bacillus species that are natural and not genetically modified. These probiotics are in the form of spores which are encapsulated in microcapsules and then weaved in the textile by Purotex® technology. Upon friction, while sleeping, these microcapsules rupture and the probiotics bacteria are released. This unexpected result may raise the hypothesis that probiotics may have a direct effect on the patient rather than acting via altering HDM allergen levels.
- *Daily vacuuming of mattresses:* This measure has shown that after 2 weeks, there was an improvement in total symptom scores such as sneezing, rhinorrhea, nasal obstruction, and itching.
- *Acaricides:* This measure has been shown to be effective in controlling the HDM antigen load in indoors and has proven to be effective in improving the VAS and overall quality of life in PAR patients with HDM sensitization. Also, no irritation or toxic effects were seen in subjects exposed to these chemicals. The acaricide studied is 0.1% Emamectin.
- *Cockroach allergy:* The cockroaches such as any other pests need food, water, and shelter to survive. By keeping a check on these basic requirements their population can be controlled. Following are the salient measures that can be deployed in their control:
    - Trash cans need to be covered tightly.
    - Eatables are to be stored in air-tight containers.
    - Dirty utensils should not be left in the sink and should be rinsed immediately so that leftover food does not remain on the utensils.
    - Food particles should be cleaned from the table tops, kitchen slabs, and stove tops by vacuuming or wet mopping on a daily basis.
    - Leaky pipes in the under-sink area should be fixed promptly.
    - Cracks in the walls are potential entry points for cockroaches and should be sealed.
    - Cockroaches baits such as gels and sticky traps are good safe and nontoxic measures.

Individual Control Measures

- *Nasal filters:* Nasal filters used during pollen season have shown benefits in reducing seasonal symptoms by decreasing the exposure to culprit pollen. They have been studied in outdoor settings, such as parks, gardens, and meadows.
- *Nasal topical microemulsions:* This is a mixture of glycerol mono-oleate, propylene glycol, polyethylene glycol 400, sesame oil, and polysorbate 80 in isotonic saline. The topical application in the nostrils did show improvement in VAS scores and quality of life among patients with both SAR and PAR, however the results were statistically not significant.

Combined Measures

A combination of environmental and individual measures have been mixed and matched in different permutations and combinations and have yielded an array of results, most of them showing improvement in symptom scores and overall quality of life, however, different subsets of patients respond differently, hence a one size fits all type of approach is yet not available and more good quality studies need to be put forth to strike the right combination for optimum symptom control in both PAR and SAR patients, thus enhancing the overall quality of life.

■ SUMMARY

- The science of prevention is more robust than before in allergic diseases, with multilevel prevention from primary to all the way to fourth prevention.
- Recent research and evidence have proven to achieve "tolerance" to inflicting antigens more effective than "avoidance" measures. Hence, AIT is deemed to be a more effective prevention modality at all levels of prevention.
- Avoidance of cigarette smoke (both passive and active) along with avoidance of indoor moisture and mold is helpful in the prevention of wheezing and asthma.
- Avoidance of dust mite allergens to prevent dust mite allergy is not recommended anymore.
- Epidemiological studies support the concept of a traditional farm environment which leads to allergy reduction in later life.
- Supplementation with vitamins, pre-, and probiotics is not detrimental but concrete evidence supporting its beneficial aspect for the prevention of allergic diseases is still lacking.
- Allergen-SIT is now gaining wide acceptance and is being implemented for milder AR as it has a disease-modifying effect if commenced early.

- Molecular advancements in allergens have led to component-resolved prophylaxis as a part of precision-based medicine tailored specifically to individual patients.
- Control measures at varied levels have proven to be successful in improving the symptom scores and overall quality of life of both SAR and PAR alike.

■ KEY POINTS

- *Importance of early intervention:* Preventive strategies for atopic diseases need to start during pregnancy and early infancy to be most effective. Primary prevention is ideal but challenging in real-world scenarios, highlighting the importance of identifying at-risk patients early through family history and close monitoring.
- *Environmental and microbial exposure:* Exposure to diverse microbiota and farm environments, owning pets such as dogs, and avoiding C-sections when possible, have shown protective effects against allergies. These exposures help in developing immune tolerance and reducing the risk of allergies.
- *Allergen-specific immunotherapy (AIT):* AIT is effective in modifying the disease course in allergic patients, particularly in those with mild AR. It is considered more beneficial than avoidance measures and is gaining acceptance for early intervention.
- *Climate change and air pollution:* Increasing air pollution and climate change are significant factors contributing to the global rise in allergic diseases. Efforts to combat these environmental issues can help reduce the prevalence of allergies.
- *Combined preventive measures:* A multifaceted approach involving environmental control (e.g., temperature and humidity control and use of air purifiers), individual measures (e.g., nasal filters), and combined strategies have been shown to improve symptom control and quality of life for patients with AR. Personalized, component-resolved prophylaxis is emerging as a precision-based preventive measure.

■ SUGGESTED READING

1. Berings M, Jult A, Vermeulen H, De Ruyck N, Derycke L, Ucar H, et al. Probiotics-impregnated bedding covers for house dust mite allergic rhinitis: a pilot randomized clinical trial. Clin Exp Allergy. 2017;47(8):1092-6.
2. Cosme-Blanco W, Arce-Ayala Y, Malinow I, Nazario S. Primary and Secondary Environmental Control Measures for Allergic Diseases. In: Mahmoudi M (Ed). Allergy and Asthma: The Basics to Best Practices. Cham: Springer; 2019. pp. 785-819.

3. Cronin C, Salzberg N, Woon Y, Wurttele JT. Primary, secondary and tertiary prevention of food allergy: current practices and future directions. Allergol Immunopathol (Madr). 2024;52(2):32-44.
4. Konradsen JR, Fujisawa T, van Hage M, Hedlin G, Hilger C, Kleine-Tebbe J, et al. Allergy to furry animals: New insights, diagnostic approaches, and challenges. J Allergy Clin Immunol. 2015;135(3):616-25. https://doi.org/10.1016/j.jaci.2014.08.026
5. Liu Y, Liu Z. Epidemiology, Prevention and Clinical Treatment of Allergic Rhinitis: More Understanding, Better Patient Care. J Clin Med. 2022;11(20):6062.
6. Manuyakorn W, Padungpak S, Luecha O, Kamchaisatian W, Sasisakulporn C, Vilaiyuk S, et al. Assessing the efficacy of a novel temperature and humidity control machine to minimize house dust mite allergen exposure and clinical symptoms in allergic rhinitis children sensitized to dust mites: a pilot study. Asian Pac J Allergy Immunol. 2015;33(2):129-35.
7. Muñoz-López F. Allergy: prevention and its problems. The fourth prevention. Allergologia Et Immunopathologia. 2002;30(4):195-8.
8. Ring J. History of Allergy: Clinical Descriptions, Pathophysiology, and Treatment. Handb Exp Pharmacol. 2022;268:3-19.
9. Tomé M, Lourenço O. Avoidance Measures for Patients with Allergic Rhinitis: A Scoping Review. Children (Basel). 2023;10(2):300.
10. Traidl-Hoffmann C, Zuberbier T, Werfel, T. Allergic Diseases – From Basic Mechanisms to Comprehensive Management and Prevention. Switzerland AG: Springer Nature; 2021.

CHAPTER 15

Evidence-based Complementary and Alternative Medicine for Allergic Rhinitis

Kashinath G Metri

■ INTRODUCTION

Allergic diseases, such as allergic bronchitis, skin allergies, food allergies, and allergic rhinitis have increased in the last 10-15 years. Any allergy, including allergic rhinitis, is an exaggerated immune reaction to a harmless stimulus, such as dust, pollen, and smoke. This type of immune reaction includes inflammation and local and systemic symptoms. There is evidence that unhealthy lifestyle and genetic predisposition contribute significantly to the development of allergic diseases by impairing immune function. An unhealthy diet, irregular sleeping habits, no or excessive physical activity, and chronic stress are the fundamental components of an unhealthy lifestyle. In the long term, an unhealthy lifestyle leads to many pathological changes in the body, such as immune dysregulation, excessive cytokine levels, insulin resistance, and autonomic dysfunction (increased sympathetic tone and lower parasympathetic tone). These chronic pathological changes in the body eventually develop into chronic diseases, such as diabetes mellitus, obesity, metabolic syndrome, autoimmune diseases, and allergic diseases. Therefore, the treatment of allergic rhinitis should include lifestyle changes. Conventional medicine plays only a limited role in the treatment of chronic diseases. In addition, it brings with its side effects. Therefore, the use of other medical systems in addition to modern medicine will be more effective. The use of complementary and alternative medicine (CAM) in the prevention and treatment of chronic diseases has increased exponentially over the last two decades. Thorough scientific research has examined the potential benefits of CAMs such as Ayurveda, yoga, homeopathy, and the Siddha system of medicine. These CAMs have been shown to be effective in reducing systemic inflammation, oxidative stress, and endocrine dysfunction.

■ AYURVEDA AND ALLERGIC RHINITIS

Ayurveda is an ancient and indigenous system of medicine. Prevention and treatment of the disease is the motto of Ayurveda. Ayurveda recognizes three energy principles in the body called "tridosha". Vata, pitta, and kapha are the tridosha **(Fig. 1)**.

A healthy state is an indication of a balanced dosha. Any imbalance in the dosha leads to disease. Thus, the treatment of any disease is the restoration of the dosha balance.

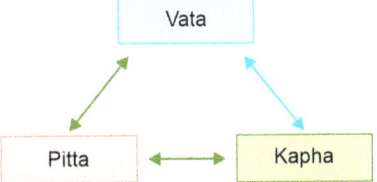

Fig. 1: Vata, pitta, and kapha are the tridosha that govern the physical and physiological activities in the body.

The tridosha balance is greatly influenced by lifestyle factors. An unhealthy diet, inadequate or excessive physical activity, mental afflictions, such as anxiety, depression, stress, hate, and worry or seasonal variations often cause imbalance in tridosha and lead to various chronic disorders.

In order to keep this tridosha in a balanced state, Ayurveda prescribes a specific lifestyle to individuals with a particular personality type (Prakriti) that consists of Dinacharya (daily regimen) and Ritucharya (seasonal regimen).

Ayurveda Perspective on Allergic Rhinitis

Having said that, any disease is imbalanced in the tridosha; allergic rhinitis is also caused by dosha imbalance. Depending on the dominant dosha involved in allergic rhinitis, symptoms may vary.

Ayurveda Treatment Approach to Allergic Disorders

According to Ayurveda, allergic rhinitis is due to an imbalance in the tridosha. Allergic rhinitis resembles to the disease *Pratishaya* mentioned in Ayurveda. Pratishaya can be caused by an imbalance of any one or combination of two or three doshas. The diagnosis of the type of Pratishaya is made on the basis of clinical features.

Allergic rhinitis can correlate with pratishaya, which the Ayurveda texts mention.

Prodromal Symptoms of Pratishaya

Symptoms such as excess sneezing, heaviness in the head, congestion in the nose and sinuses, itching sensation in the nose, change in voice, anorexia, and excess salivation are the prodromal symptoms of pratishaya. These can be considered symptoms that occur before acute episodes of allergic rhinitis. Depending on dominant dosha involvement, these symptoms may vary from person to person.

Pratishaya is a condition with tridosha imbalance in the upper respiratory tract. Depending on dosha involvement, the symptoms of pratishaya vary from person to person.

Based on dosha involvement, there are five types of pratishaya described here.

Vata dosha dominant Pratishaya: In this type, vata is the dominant dosha.

Symptoms—Excess sneezing, nasal block, scanty and watery nasal secretion, dryness in the nose, nasal cavity and throat, headache, and change in the voice. The allergic rhinitis in these symptoms can be attributed to vata-dominant pratishaya, which can be treated accordingly.

Pitta dosha dominant Pratishaya: In this type, the pitta is the dominant dosha.

Symptoms: Burning sensation in the nose, yellow-colored discharge, boils in the nose, dry mouth and palate, excess thirst, and fever.

Kapha dosha dominant Pratishaya: In this type, the kapha is the dominant dosha.

White and thick mucus secretion, heaviness in the head, nasal congestion, edema around the eyes, itching sensation in the throat, nose, and palate region, stiffness in the neck, nausea, vomiting, lethargy, and anorexia.

All three doshas dominant Pratishaya: In this type, all three doshas get aggravated. This type of pratishaya often subsides on itself without any treatment and frequently comes in acute episodes.

Raktaj Pratishaya: It is a severe and rare form of pratishaya associated with nasal breeding, eye redness, and halitosis.

In clinical practice, patients with allergic rhinitis exhibit different groups of symptoms. According to Ayurveda, these variations in the symptoms are due to the dominant dosha involved in the manifestation of allergic rhinitis. Hence, the treatment of allergic rhinitis is based on the dominant dosha engaged in the allergic rhinitis.

Treatment of Allergic Rhinitis According to Ayurveda

Ayurveda is a form of lifestyle medicine that prescribes lifestyle modification and herbal medications. The following lifestyle modifications are specified in the treatment of allergic rhinitis.

Apathya (contraindications): During acute episodes of allergic rhinitis, patients should avoid baths, exposure to cold and heat, suppression of natural calls, and consuming excess liquid. Should not indulge in heated arguments, debates, and should not grief. Patients with allergic rhinitis should avoid food items, such as cool drinks, curd, milk, and refined carbs.

Pathya (indications): Ginger, garlic, honey, snake guard, warm water, old grains, drumstick, porridge and rice soups, and mung dal. Fresh and warm food mixed with healthy fats is recommended. Ghee consumption is beneficial.

Ayurveda is an individualized system of practice based on individual assessments such as the basic and disturbed status of *doshas (prakriti and vikriti), agni, dhatu,* and many other parameters. Hence, the clinician selects a combination of medications, such as *Haridra Khanda, Chyavanprash, Sitopaladi Churna, and Vasa Avaleha,* for allergic disorders after assessing each case. For chronic allergic conditions, *Ayurveda* recommends *Panchakarma* (systemic purificatory therapies), which is to be administered under the supervision of an *Ayurveda* physician (Patel et al. 2013).

Ayurveda recommends panchakarma procedures in the treatment of allergic rhinitis. The different types of panchakarma therapies are recommended based on the dominant dosha involved in allergic rhinitis.

Snehana (oleation therapy) and Swedana (sudation therapy), which are the preparatory practices of panchakarma, help treat allergic rhinitis.

Ayurveda nasya chikitsa (nasal medication): Nasya is a popular therapy intervention in Ayurveda. In this therapy, Ayurveda medications are administered through nasal route **(Fig. 2)**. Nasya therapy is used to treat a variety of health conditions including allergic rhinitis. Different types of medicated oils or decoctions are used for nasya therapy to treat allergic rhinitis. Anu taila and ghee are widely recommended for nasya in allergic rhinitis.

Ayurveda medications: Medications, such as Bhallataka Parpati, Bhallatakasava, Chitrakadi Vati, Sanjivani Vati, Sitopaladi Churna,

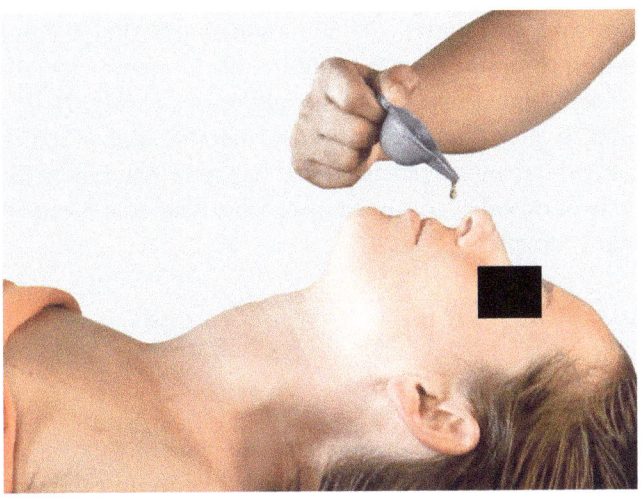

Fig. 2: The demonstration of Ayurveda nasya procedure.

Talisapatradi Churna, Chyavanprash, and Vasavaleha are found to be effective allergic rhinitis.

During acute episodes Tribhuvankirti rasa and Nagavati are recommended.

Scientific Evidence of Ayurveda in Allergic Rhinitis

Clinical trials on nasya therapy have shown positive effects on nasal allergy. Thirty-seven patients with nasal allergy received Anu taila nasya therapy daily for 2 months in a study. Postintervention, there was a significant decrease in nasal allergy symptoms, total leukocyte count (TLC), absolute eosinophil count (AEC), neutrophils, and lymphocytes.

■ YOGA

Yoga is a science of mind-body practices. Yoga helps to build a positive attitude and improves physical and mental health. Recently, yoga has become a popular intervention in the treatment and management of various chronic health problems, including allergic conditions, such as asthma and allergic rhinitis.

Allergic Rhinitis According to Yoga

Yoga recognizes every individual as a Jivatma (individual consciousness). Jivatma is made up of five components called Panchakosha. They are (1) annamaya kosha, the physical anatomical component made of chemicals (pockets of particles, atoms, cells, tissues, and organ systems), (2) pranamaya kosha, the vital body, the biomagnetic field responsible for all physiological functions (movement and reproduction), (3) manomaya kosha, the mind (perception and emotions), (4) Vijñānamaya kosha, the intellectual discriminating component of the mind, and (5) anandamaya kosha, the causal bliss field (stable, rested, and thoughtless state) **(Fig. 3)**.

According to yoga, allergy is a peripheral manifestation of ādhi (emotional imbalances in the manomaya kosha) that begins in the mind and shows up as immune hyperreactivity in annamaya kosha. Ādhi also diverts the person from a healthy lifestyle.

Techniques of Yoga-based Lifestyle Change for Allergic Disorders

Diet Modification

Food significantly influences the mental state. According to yoga, there are three types of foods: (1) the food that makes the mind calm and stable is called "sattva"; (2) the food that makes the mind excited, passionate, and

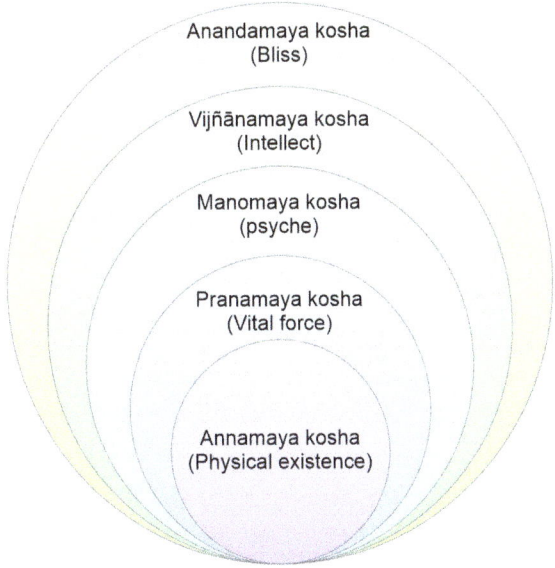

Fig. 3: Panchakosha—the five components of human existence.

aggressive is called "rajasic" food; and (3) the food that causes drowsiness/laziness is called "tamasic" food. Thus, the recommended sattvic food for health is nutritious, simple, wholesome, freshly cooked, and satmya (suitable) foods consumed in moderate quantities (Bhagavad Gita). Avoid processed, deep-fried, refined, heavily spiced foods considered rajasic, and fermented, preserved, or stale foods as tamasic. Yoga and Ayurveda also suggest that persons with allergic diseases should follow sattvic diet and avoid the food that aggravates the allergy symptoms. Identify the allergens in the food and prevent them initially, but develop tolerance to use healthy food items later as the system becomes more stable through regular yoga practices.

Kriyas—The Yogic Cleansing Techniques

Kriyas refer to techniques of cleansing the internal passages. The recommended cleaning techniques (kriyas) for allergic rhinitis include jala neti and sutra neti to cleanse the nasopharyngeal tract. They help to clear the internal passages in the nose and nasal cavity and reduce hypersensitivity of the nasal mucosa, resulting in better tolerance to harmless external substances.

Jala Neti

Jala neti—nasal irrigation using warm saline water: Jala neti is widely practiced and popular kriya in yoga.

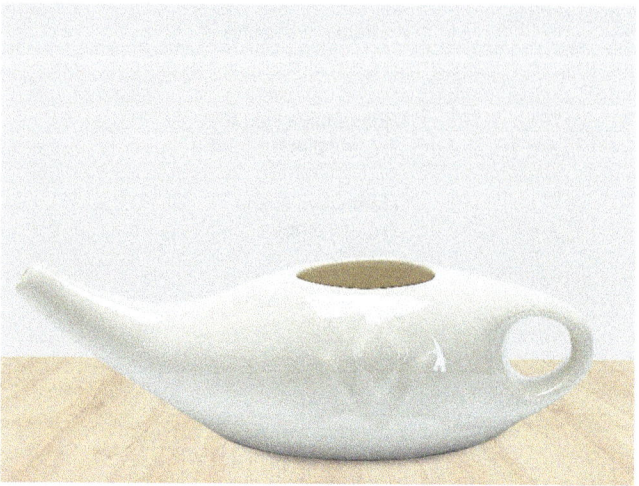

Fig. 4: Neti pot.

Procedure: Jala neti and sutra neti should be practiced on an empty stomach early in the morning. Before the practice of jala neti, one should ensure no nasal congestion (free air flow in both nostrils). Nasal congestion can be removed by performing kapalabhati (forceful and dynamic exhalation by flapping the abdomen—2 × 40 strokes/minute) **(Fig. 4)**.

Jala neti is performed using lukewarm (39°C) saline water (2.5 g NaCl/500 m water) in a neti pot. One should stand straight, bend forward, and tilt the neck to the right side. Nasal irrigation is done by inserting the neti pot's nozzle into the right nostril. During nasal irrigation, one should breathe from the mouth. After the right nostril, repeat the procedure for the left nostril. After completion, one should perform kapalabhati to drain out the left saline water in the nostril **(Fig. 5)**.

One should avoid jala neti during an acute episode of allergic rhinitis, acute sinusitis, acute exacerbation of asthma, nasal polyps, and severe form of the deviated nasal septum.

Sutra Neti

This kriya involves the insertion of a rubber catheter in the nostril through the nasal cavity, which is taken out from the mouth through the posterior nasal orifice. Both ends of the catheter are held with fingers, and a gentle massage is done by smoothly pulling the catheter back-and-forth 5–10 times **(Figs. 6 and 7)**.

Patients with allergic rhinitis should practice these kriyas under the supervision of a trained yoga therapist twice a week for a minimum of 3 months to observe changes.

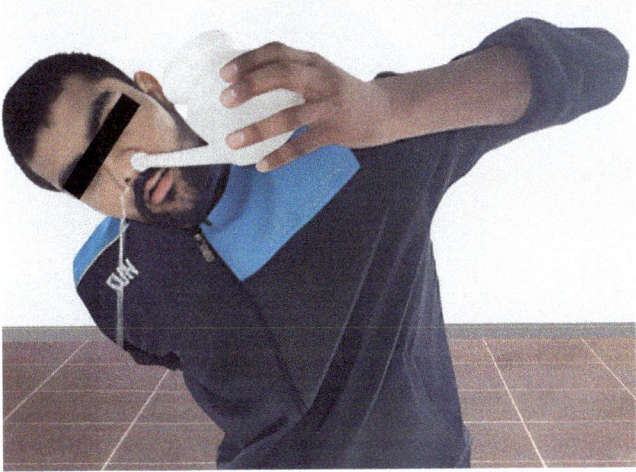

Fig. 5: Demonstration of jala neti practice.

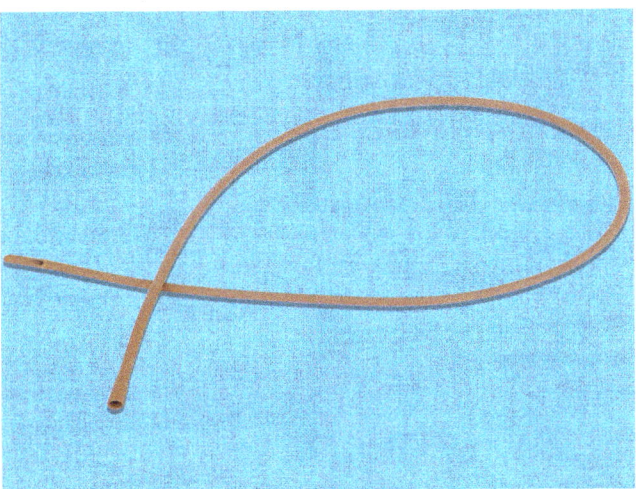

Fig. 6: Sutra neti catheter.

Asana (Yoga Postures)

Asana practice involves mindfulness stretching followed by relaxation. Asana practice helps to improve autonomic dysfunction and reduce cortisol, and it has immunomodulation property, which helps to reduce inflammatory cytokines and systemic inflammation. The list of yoga practices that are useful for treating allergic rhinitis is listed in **Table 1**.

These yoga practices should be performed on an empty stomach or 2–21/2 hours after a meal. Yoga postures should be done slowly with deep,

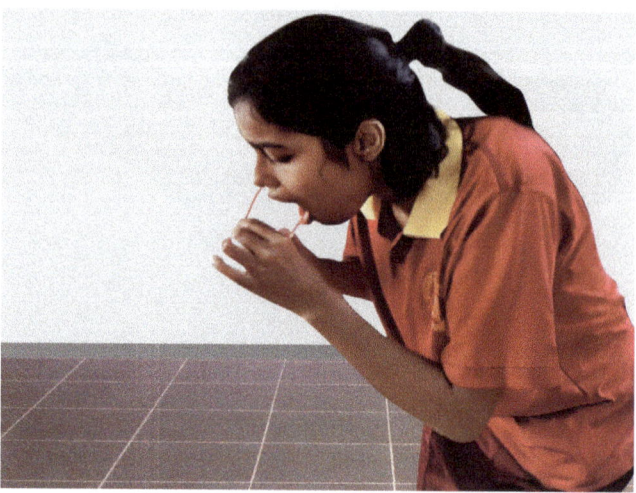

Fig. 7: Demonstration of sutra neti practice.

TABLE 1: The list of yoga practices for allergic disorders.	
Practice	**Duration—60 minutes**
Loosening practices	10 minutes
Quick relaxation technique (QRT)	
Breathing practices	15 minutes
Prasarita hasta swasah (hands in and out breathing)	
Hands stretch breathing	
Vyaghra swasah (tiger breathing)	
Ankle stretch breathing	
Straight leg raising breathing	
Setu bandhasana breathing (breathing in bridge pose)	
Bhujangasana breathing (breathing in cobra pose)	
Asanas	20 minutes
Tadasana (straight pose)	
Trikonasana (triangle pose)	
Padahastasana (hand-feet pose)	
Ardha kati chakrasana (half-waist pose)	
Bhunamanasana	
Setu bandhasana	
Markatasana	
Ustrasana (camel pose)	
Shavasana (corpse pose)	

Contd...

Contd...

Practice	Duration—60 minutes
Deep relaxation technique (DRT)	10 minutes
Pranayama (yogic breathing practices)	5 minutes
Bhastrika pranayama (bellows breath)	
Nadi shodhana pranayama (alternate nostril breathing)	
Bhramari pranayama (humming)	

slow, and conscious breathing. Do not strain; try to attempt the pose easily (it is okay if a final/perfect posture is not possible). After reaching the final pose, one should hold the pose with their capacity with normal breathing.

Pranayama (Yogic Breathing)

Pranayama is slow-paced, mindful breathing. There are various types of breathing practices according to yoga, such as alternate nostril breathing (nadi shodhana pranayama), left nostril breathing (Chandra nadi pranayama), and right nostril breathing (Surya nadi pranayama).

The patients with allergic rhinitis should practice pranayama, such as nadi shodhana pranayama, Bhramari pranayama, Ujjayi pranayama, and Vibhagiya pranayama. Cooling pranayamas, such as sheetali, sitkari, sadanta, and Chandra nadi pranayama should be avoided.

Meditation

Meditation is a yogic mental practice that involves the practice of mental focusing on a meditative object/thought/mantra, etc., followed by defocusing. Meditations, such as OM, mindfulness, vipassana, and cyclic meditation are recommended for allergic rhinitis. Meditation is associated with decreased inflammatory cytokines, catecholamine, cortisol, and sympathetic overactivity. Thus, meditation may help in reducing frequency and severity of acute episodes of allergic rhinitis by reducing inflammation **(Table 1)**.

Yoga and Immune Modulation

Rigors scientific investigations have confirmed the benefits of yoga practice in improving immune function. Yoga helps immune modulation. Yoga reduces inflammatory cytokines, and increases natural killer (NK) cell number and immune cell activity. Clinical trials have shown the positive role of yoga in immune-compromised conditions, such as human immunodeficiency virus (HIV), tuberculosis, and cancer. Yoga intervention demonstrated the increase in NK-cell activity and T lymphocytes, CD4, CD8, and NK-cell count and reduced inflammatory cytokines, such as interleukin-1 (IL-1), IL-2,

IL-6, and tumor necrosis factor-α (TNF-α). Further, psychological factors, such as anxiety, depression, stress, and mood, which are known to affect immune function reduced after yoga intervention. Yoga brings the immune modulation by reducing catecholamines, cortisol, and inflammatory cytokines via downregulating hypothalamic-pituitary-adrenal (HPA) axis hyperactivity and improving the vagal tone.

Yoga in Allergic Rhinitis

Studies have demonstrated the benefits of yoga in allergic rhinitis. An randomized controlled trial (RCT) on 8-week hatha yoga intervention (3 times/week) among 27 allergic rhinitis patients has shown significant improvement in clinical symptoms of rhinitis and cytokine profiles. Another study on 51 healthy volunteers and 51 allergic rhinitis patients who received 3 months of hath yoga intervention showed a significant decrease in nasal airway resistance. It increased forced vital capacity and a nonsignificant increase in FEV1. Further, mental health measures and sinonasal outcome tests also improved significantly. Following yoga practice, the positive changes in allergic rhinitis may be attributed to immune modulation by reducing inflammatory cytokines, improved circulation to the nasal mucosa, and decreased hypersensitivity of the nasal mucosa. Persons with allergic rhinitis are recommended regular yoga practices consisting of loosening practices, yoga postures, and yoga breathing practices (listed in **Table 1**) a minimum of three times a week, and jala neti practice a minimum of twice a week for a minimum of 3 months.

■ BEHAVIOR THERAPIES IN ALLERGIC RHINITIS

Recently, behavior therapies, such as cognitive behavioral therapy (CBT) have gained popularity in the management of chronic disorders. These therapies help the patients to recognize their health conditions, develop positive and realistic perception about the disease condition, and help to develop positive coping strategies to overcome the distress associated with the ongoing health issues.

In allergic rhinitis, patient should be educated about the disease and its symptoms. The patient should be assured that the symptoms can be minimized by making few changes in the lifestyle, such as eating habits and avoiding AC, cold should be educated about how mental afflictions, such as anger, distress, and anxiety contribute to exacerbation of allergic rhinitis.

Most often, the allergic rhinitis leads to distress and depression and it significantly affect the daily to day activities and patient's quality of life. Behavior interventions such as CBT help to develop mental well-being by reducing distress and depression.

SUMMARY

Allergic rhinitis is a chronic health condition. Unhealthy lifestyle is considered to be an important factor in the cause, maintenance, and aggravation allergic rhinitis. Complementary and alternative therapies such as Ayurveda and Yoga recommend a healthy lifestyle which includes diet modification, specific yoga practice, and herbal medications in the treatment of allergic rhinitis. Scientific evidence suggests that both Ayurveda and Yoga therapy have a potential role in the treatment and management of allergic rhinitis.

KEY POINTS

- *Holistic approach to allergic rhinitis:* The chapter emphasizes the importance of a holistic approach in treating allergic rhinitis, integrating lifestyle changes, and CAM therapies such as Ayurveda and yoga. This approach addresses both the symptoms and underlying causes of allergic conditions.
- *Ayurveda's Tridosha theory:* Ayurveda attributes allergic rhinitis to an imbalance in the three doshas (vata, pitta, and kapha). Treatment involves restoring dosha balance through lifestyle modifications, dietary changes, and specific herbal medications tailored to the individual's dosha constitution and imbalances.
- *Efficacy of nasya therapy:* Nasya therapy, an Ayurvedic practice of administering medicated oils or decoctions through the nasal route, has shown significant benefits in clinical trials for reducing symptoms and inflammatory markers in nasal allergies.
- *Yoga's role in immune modulation:* Yoga practices, including asanas (postures), pranayama (breathing techniques), and kriyas (cleansing techniques), have been scientifically shown to improve immune function, reduce inflammatory cytokines, and enhance overall mental and physical health, thus benefiting those with allergic rhinitis.
- *Behavioral therapies and mental health:* Behavioral therapies, such as CBT, play a crucial role in managing allergic rhinitis by helping patients develop positive coping strategies, reducing distress and depression, and improving their quality of life. These therapies complement the physical treatments provided by Ayurveda and yoga.

SUGGESTED READING

1. Achilles N, Mösges R. Nasal saline irrigations for the symptoms of acute and chronic rhinosinusitis. Curr Allergy Asthma Rep. 2013;13:229-35.
2. Balkrishna A, Rana M, Mishra S, Srivastava D, Bhardwaj R, Singh S, et al. Incredible Combination of Lifestyle Modification and Herbal Remedies for Polycystic Ovarian Syndrome Management. Evid Based Complement Alternat Med. 2023;2023:3705508.

3. Bhavanani AB. Understanding the science of Yoga. Int Sci Yoga J. 2011;1:334-44.
4. Chellaa R, Soumya MS, Inbaraj G, Nayar R, Saidha PK, Menezes VH, et al. Impact of Hatha Yoga on the Airway Resistances in Healthy Individuals and Allergic Rhinitis Patients. Indian J Otolaryngol Head Neck Surg. 2019;71(Suppl 3):1748-56.
5. Gupta V, Khanna K, Gupta RK. A study on the street food dimensions and its effects on consumer attitude and behavioural intentions. Tour Rev. 2018;73(3):374-88.
6. Hankey A. The scientific value of Ayurveda. J Altern Complement Med. 2005;11(2):221-5.
7. Meera S, Rani MV, Sreedhar C, Robin DT. A review on the therapeutic effects of Neti Kriya with special reference to Jala Neti. J Ayurveda Integr Med. 2020;11(2):185-9.
8. Metri KG, Vedanthan PK. Role of Yoga and Ayurveda in the Management of Allergic Disorders. In: Vedanthan PK, Nelson HS, Bever HV, Murali MR (Eds). Textbook of Diagnostic and Therapeutic Procedures in Allergy. Boca Raton: CRC Press; 2024. pp. 328-41.
9. Morais P, Quaresma C, Vigário R, Quintão C. Electrophysiological effects of mindfulness meditation in a concentration test. Med Biol Eng Comput. 2021;59(4):759-73.
10. Nagendra HR, Nagarathna R. An integrated approach of yoga therapy for bronchial asthma: a 3–54-month prospective study. J Asthma. 1986;23(3):123-37.
11. Newcombe S. Yoga and meditation as a health intervention. In: Newcombe S, O'Brien-Kop K (Eds). Routledge Handbook of Yoga and Meditation Studies. London: Taylor & Francis; 2020.
12. Prinster T. Yoga for Cancer: a guide to managing side effects, boosting immunity, and improving recovery for Cancer survivors. New York: Simon and Schuster; 2014.

Futuristic View

Rupali Patil Jain

■ INTRODUCTION

Allergic rhinitis (AR) is a type 1 hypersensitivity reaction mediated by immunoglobulin E (IgE) responses to certain inhaled allergens. It is associated with a lot of comorbidities and affects the quality of life (QOL) even though it is not a life-threatening disease. It can also exacerbate diseases such as chronic obstructive pulmonary disease (COPD) and other respiratory illnesses. Mild-to-moderate AR patients are treated with pharmacotherapy which in the long term can have side effects and rebound congestion. If complete allergen avoidance cannot be achieved or if immunotherapy has not been effective or contraindicated due to some reason, or if patients are sensitized to multiple allergens, we need newer therapeutic molecules to treat this. Several studies have been going on to develop some oral, intranasal, and alternative forms of immunotherapy other than the conventional ones such as subcutaneous immunotherapy (SCIT) and sublingual immunotherapy (SLIT). Some of them are in phase 2/phase 3 trials. These newer molecules have been discussed here.

■ HYDROXYPROPYL METHYLCELLULOSE POWDER

Allergic rhinitis symptoms are triggered when nasal mucosa is exposed to pollen, spores, occupational inhalants, and pollutants. Hydroxypropyl methylcellulose (HPMC) in powder form is a derivative of cellulose. Three in vitro studies were conducted for pollens, dust mites, and pollutants, and in vivo studies on rats. A specially designed patented delivery system has been made to deliver it into the nose as a microcrystalline powder. When insufflated nasally, it swells and forms a gel barrier against inhaled allergenic agents and pollutants reducing the nasal symptoms and enhancing the effects of intranasal medications used for local treatment. HPMC being hygroscopic in nature swells as soon as it comes in contact with moisture in the nasal cavity as well as moisture in nasal air. No particle size of PHMC was <1.9 µm, so none of the particles would reach the alveoli and instead would be swallowed as they would be trapped in the pharynx. So, a targeted deposition in the nasal cavity could be achieved.

In vitro studies showed that in the absence of a barrier, house dust mite absorption was 100% after 60 minutes but with a barrier, it was 0.76% after

15 minutes and 28.1% after 360 minutes. Pollen absorption (Amb a 1 used in this study) was 3.06% and pollutant absorption was reduced by 94%. In vivo studies on rats showed no evidence of inflammation in target organs, such as lungs, liver, and brain at 1, 24, and 48 hours after challenge. There were no significantly different changes in heart rate, arterial oxygen saturation, and in mean arterial pressure. A tolerable intake for ingestion of PHMC by humans of 5 mg/kg/day is accepted. It is available under the brand name Nasaleze.

■ LIPID MICROEMULSION

Topical nasal microemulsion made of glycerol esters is another barrier protection method to avoid contact with allergens. Its mechanism of action consists of creating a lipid coating that spreads over the surface of the nasal mucosa. A lipid barrier is created which prevents allergens from being deposited on the nasal mucosa. The formulation of the topical microemulsion consists of glycerol monooleate, propylene glycol, polyethylene glycol 400, sesame oil, polysorbate 80, sodium chloride 0.9%, menthol, eucalyptus oil, and water. A study was conducted to compare its efficacy in patients with AR caused by pollen allergen. It was seen that intranasal administration of small volumes of a microemulsion twice daily reduced overall nasal symptoms when administered during the pollen season. This was compared to an isotonic saline which was used as a placebo. These microemulsions are useful options for reducing symptoms of seasonal rhinitis.

■ RESVERATROL

Reactive oxygen species (ROS) are generated by epithelial cells and dendritic cells (DCs) when they come in contact with allergens or particulate matter. ROS contributes to the induction of Th2 responses through various cellular and molecular mechanisms. Thioredoxin-interacting protein (TXNIP) plays a crucial role in the production of ROS. Resveratrol, a TXNIP inhibitor, can inhibit ROS production and reduce oxidative stress.

In a study conducted on ovalbumin (OVA)-induced AR murine model, OVA was given in injectable form intraperitoneally on days 1, 8, and 15. From days 22 to 29, OVA was given intranasally daily. Resveratrol was administered intranasally from days 22 to 29. Sneezing and nose rubbing were significantly decreased. OVA-specific IgE, eosinophil numbers in nasal tissue, serum and nasal lavage fluid cytokine levels, prostaglandin D2 (PGD2), leukotriene C4 (LTC4), eosinophil cationic protein (ECP), interleukin 4 (IL4), IL5, IL6, IL33, tumor necrosis factor-α (TNF-α), TXNIP mRNA levels, and malondialdehyde (MDA) levels were diminished. The superoxide dismutase (SOD) level was elevated.

Resveratrol may be a promising new therapy for AR.

SODIUM PYRUVATE

Higher levels of ROS can lead to various harmful changes in the airway lining, such as increased lipid peroxidation, heightened airway reactivity, greater sensitivity and secretions in the nasal mucosa, generation of molecules that attract immune cells, increased permeability of blood vessels, and congestion. Sodium pyruvate, a natural antioxidant produced within the body, plays a significant role in safeguarding cells against oxidative stress, potentially shielding organs from radical-induced harm. Moreover, sodium pyruvate can inhibit the interaction between nitric oxide and hydrogen peroxide, which otherwise forms the harmful peroxynitrite compound; both of these compounds are elevated in AR, contributing to inflammation and congestion.

Five human clinical trials were done. Out of which first and second were phase 1, open-labeled, baseline-controlled trial, third was double-blind, computer randomized, placebo-controlled phase 2 and 3, fourth was open-labeled, placebo-controlled phase 2 and 3, and fifth was double-blind, placebo-controlled phase 2 and 3 in which sodium pyruvate was given to AR patients intranasally.

Patients exhibited notable reductions in levels of proinflammatory cytokines and oxidative molecules, such as IL6, IL8, monocyte chemoattractant protein-1, and hydrogen peroxide. Comparing nasal inflammation scores to those of the control group treated with a placebo or receiving no treatment initially, it was found that all patients experienced a decrease in nasal inflammation and congestion. Despite these positive outcomes, additional double-blind, placebo-controlled studies are necessary moving forward. Given its potential efficacy in lessening nasal inflammation, sodium pyruvate may also prove beneficial for conditions, such as COPD, pulmonary fibrosis, coronavirus disease 2019 (COVID-19), and long COVID, as these conditions often involve nasal inflammation.

PF-03654746 WITH FEXOFENADINE

Nasal congestion due to AR results from the combined effects of venous vessel dilation leading to engorgement and tissue edema. In patients with rhinitis, vascular tone, which is regulated by sympathetic neural control, is defective, while plasma protein leakage occurs due to histamine released from mast cells acting on H1 receptors on the vascular endothelium. H3 receptors function as inhibitory autoreceptors/heteroreceptors that regulate the release of neuroactive and vasoactive mediators. Nasal H3 receptors may play a role in mediating histamine's effects in patients with AR. PF-03654746, a potent H3 receptor antagonist, has been demonstrated to block H3 receptor agonist-induced decreases in cyclic adenosine monophosphate (AMP) accumulation in vitro, and it also exhibits inverse agonist activity. This compound shows significant selectivity for H3 receptors over H1, H2, and H4 receptors.

A study explored the effects of the potent H3 antagonist PF-03654746 in combination with an oral H1 receptor antagonist on patients' symptoms and acoustic rhinometry responses to nasal allergen challenges. This study was a randomized, double-blinded, double-dummy, placebo-controlled, four-way crossover study involving subjects with a documented history of Ragweed pollen seasonal AR. Minimal cross-sectional area and nasal volume were assessed using rhinomanometry, and nasal symptoms were measured on a 0-5 scale, with the number of sneezes also counted. A nasal allergen challenge was performed using Ragweed extract (Amb a 1). The 10 mg dose of PF-03654746 plus fexofenadine significantly reduced nasal congestion symptoms. Rhinorrhea and sneeze counts were also reduced. The H3 receptor antagonist class shows potential benefits in treating AR when combined with an effective H1 receptor antagonist. However, certain side effects, such as insomnia, disorientation, anorexia, and feeling jittery necessitate larger studies.

■ SETIPIPRANT

Prostaglandin D2 is a proinflammatory mediator that influences the inflammatory cascade underlying AR through two cell surface receptors: PTGDR1 and the CRTH2 (also known as PTGDR2). When PGD2 binds to CRTH2, which is expressed on key effector cells in the allergic response cascade, it initiates a series of humoral and cellular immune reactions. These actions collectively result in eosinophilia, tissue damage, and tissue remodeling.

Setipiprant is an orally active tetrahydropyridoindole derivative and a selective CRTH2 antagonist. It inhibits the action of eosinophils and basophils and reduces cytokine secretion. Phase 2 and phase 3 prospective, randomized, double-blind, placebo-controlled, and active-referenced clinical trials found that setipiprant effectively alleviated symptoms of seasonal AR at a dose of 1,000 mg/day. The drug was well tolerated with dry mouth being the only reported side effect.

■ PHOSPHODIESTERASE INHIBITOR—ROFLUMILAST

Phosphodiesterase 4 (PDE4) inhibitors exert anti-inflammatory activity by blocking the degradation of cyclic adenosine monophosphate which is present in lymphocytes, eosinophils, neutrophils, and monocytes thus leading to an attenuated release of histamine, leukotrienes, and cytokines. Roflumilast is a PDE4 inhibitor that exerts anti-inflammatory activity in effector cells as shown in in vivo and in vitro studies. Two 250 mg tablets and a placebo were given to subjects. A controlled antigen challenge was performed on 7 consecutive days in each study period by spraying two puffs of the pollen suspension in each nostril. 5 and 30 minutes after each allergen provocation, symptoms, such as sneezing, obstruction, and rhinorrhea were evaluated on a visual analog scale and rhinometry was performed. Roflumilast provided greater improvement than placebo. It was safe and well tolerated. Adverse events reported were headache and dizziness. However, this study was performed on a small number of subjects, so further studies are required to prove the efficacy of roflumilast in patients with AR.

ALLERGOIDS

The structure of the allergen molecules can be altered or chemically modified by treatment with glutaraldehyde or formalin. This reduces the IgE-binding epitopes which makes the treatment safer. These modified allergens are called "allergoids." In a study conducted in Germany, long-term effects of pollen allergoid tyrosine adsorbed SCIT on AR and asthma were seen. SCIT allergoids allowed fast up-dosing with a good safety profile. It was well studied in controlled, intermittent, and mild persistent asthma. The study period was of four allergy seasons. Three authorized allergoids that contained grass or tree pollen were included in the study. One was tyrosine adsorbed and two were aluminum hydroxide adjuvated allergoids. Patients of age 5–65 years, who met all the criteria, were included in the study. They received at least one prescription of an AR medication. 5,959 patients were included who had a follow-up of 2 years. Each allergen immunotherapy (AIT) had a matched control group. After the AIT treatment was completed, the impact on AR progression was measured by symptomatic AR medication prescription in the follow-up period and was compared to the pretreatment period. When compared to the control group, 27.8% of patients treated with allergoids did not receive prescriptions for treatment of AR symptoms.

LOW-LEVEL LASER THERAPY

In an animal study, low-level laser therapy (LLLT) was irradiated into the intranasal cavity of an OVA albumin-induced AR mouse model. It proved effective in inhibiting IgE and IL4.

A randomized, double-blind, placebo-controlled study was designed to evaluate the effects of LLLT. Participants suffering from perennial AR, >19 years of age, suffering from mild-to-moderate symptoms and a proven positive skin prick test, with any gender or ethnicity, and who consented to the study were recruited. LLLT device and sham treatment device similar to the LLLT device were randomly allocated which was computer generated. Neither the physician nor the patients were aware of the list. 1 month prior all the medications were stopped.

Low-level laser therapy improved the symptoms and QOL significantly at the end of the 4-week treatment. Though the mechanism of LLLT has not been fully understood, the animal models showed that there was induction of interleukin-10 (IL-10), reduction in expression of macrophage inflammatory protein 2 and TNF and there was local reduction in IL-5. LLLT can inhibit TNF-α, cyclooxygenase-2, prostaglandin E2, and IL-1 beta.

■ FEL D1 CHAIN 2 GENOME-EDITED CATS

Cat is the most common source of mammalian allergen with symptoms that range from rhinoconjunctivitis to asthma. Cat allergen is ubiquitous, and can remain airborne for hours with minimal disturbance as the particle size which carries cat allergens can be very small. It takes a few months for cat allergens to reduce after the cat is removed from the home. Cat allergen is a very sticky protein, difficult to remove from carpets and clothes. Fel D1–Fel D8 are the cat allergens of which Fel D1 is the major allergen. Fel D1 is composed of two genes CH1 and CH2, linked via three disulfide bonds.

In a study conducted, the cloning of CH2 genome-edited cats which can be hypoallergenic using the CRISPR (clustered regularly interspaced short palindromic repeats)-Cas 9 gene system was reported. To edit the CH2 genome, single guide RNAs (sgRNAs) which contained C2 1 and C2 2 were designed to target the CH2 after confirming the CH2 sequence. Out of C@ 1 and C2 2, C@ 1 was selected and the mRNA of C2 1 and Cas 9 were transcribed in vitro which had to be microinjected into the feline zygotes. After microinjection, these 20 embryos were transferred into the pseudopregnant recipient female cats out of which only one cat gave birth to two kittens. The first and second kittens were mosaically and heterozygously mutated respectively in the CH2 genome. After attaining sexual maturity, these both cats were mated so as to produce CH2 homozygous genome-edited cats. Six new kittens were delivered. One male kitten was homozygous mutated in its CH2 genome and the other three male cats were heterozygously modified in their CH2 genome. A CH2 homozygous genome-edited cat was successfully cloned from a male cat using cytoplasm injection cloning technology which was confirmed by microsatellite analysis. Enzyme-linked immunosorbent assay (ELISA) was performed to investigate the levels of Fel D1 in the saliva and fur of two parent cats with their newborn kitten. This was compared to a wild-type cat. Data demonstrated the CH2 genome-edited cats showed exceptionally low levels of Fel D1.

■ INTRALYMPHATIC IMMUNOTHERAPY

Subcutaneous immunotherapy can cause some serious anaphylactic reactions. It requires 30–80 injections over a period of 3–5 years. So, alternative routes of giving immunotherapy have been studied. Out of which one is the intralymphatic route under ultrasound guidance. It was given in three doses with an interval of 4 weeks between doses. The allergen is directly delivered to B and T cells within the lymph nodes. It induces a stronger cytotoxic T-cell response and higher immunogenicity than other routes. In a monocentric open-labeled trial, after giving SCIT and intralymphatic injections in inguinal nodes, patients were evaluated at intervals of 4 months, 1 year, and 3 years by various tests. These tests were nasal provocation, skin prick testing, IgE measurements, and symptom scores. Intralymphatic injections increased tolerance to nasal provocation with pollen already within 4 months. Tolerance was long-lasting. Symptoms were ameliorated, and skin prick test reactivity and serum-specific IgE were reduced. There were fewer adverse events than SCIT, compliance was enhanced and the procedure was less painful than venous puncture. Treatment time was reduced from 3 years to 8 weeks.

■ EPICUTANEOUS IMMUNOTHERAPY

The epidermis of the skin contains a high number of antigen-presenting cells (APCs) such as Langerhans cells and a nonvascularized epithelium. Several placebo-controlled clinical trials have shown that the epicutaneous route can be an ideal route for immunotherapy. The keratinocytes can be activated by physical irritation. Epithelial damage increases keratinocyte expression of molecules, such as IL-1α, IL-6, and TNF-α, skewing the immune response toward Th1 type response. A proinflammatory environment is created. As this is a needle-free form of immunotherapy, it would be beneficial for children.

■ INTRADERMAL IMMUNOTHERAPY

Dermis contains a high density of dermal DCs that act as APCs. A proinflammatory response is carried out after the APCs carry the allergens. The regulatory T cell and B cell-mediated immune response triggers a shift from a Th2 cytokine response to a Th1 response. This shift causes the release of transforming growth factor-β (TGF-β), interferon-γ (IFN-γ), and IL-10, leading to allergen-specific immune tolerance. Consequently, there is a reduction in IgE levels and an increase in the release of immunoglobulin G4 (IgG4) and immunoglobulin A (IgA)-blocking antibodies. The ability of DCs to migrate through lymphatic vessels to skin-draining lymph nodes and induce regulatory T (Treg) cells suggests that the intradermal route may offer an advantage and enhance the efficacy of AIT. This route may facilitate a reduction in allergen dosage and shorten the treatment duration.

■ INTRATONSILLAR IMMUNOTHERAPY

A randomized double-blind, placebo-controlled clinical trial was conducted on 80 patients sensitized to house dust mites. These patients received six intratonsillar injections of either HDM extract or saline (as a placebo) over 3 months. The injections included one of 1,000 standardized quality units (SQ-U), two of 3,000 SQ-U, and three of 10,000 SQ-U, administered by ENT surgeons at the inferior pole of the palatine tonsils on both sides using a 1 mL syringe with a 0.45 × 16 mm needle, injected 2–3 mm deep. The side effects noted at the injection site included hemorrhage, dry mouth, sore throat, earache, and cutaneous pruritus.

The total nasal symptom score (TNSS), the visual analog scale of nasal symptoms, combined symptom and medication score, QOL questionnaire, and serum allergen-specific IgG4 to *Dermatophagoides pteronyssinus* were monitored at baseline, and at 3, 6, and 12 months after the treatment was completed. The TNSS in the active group significantly improved compared to the placebo group at 3 months post-treatment. However, there was no significant difference in TNSS between the active and placebo groups at 6 and 12 months post-treatment, although the difference at 12 months was statistically significant.

The Mini Rhinoconjunctivitis Quality of Life Questionnaire (RQLQ) scores significantly decreased at 3 and 12 months post-treatment in the active group compared to the placebo group. There were no significant changes in the wheal surface area in the skin prick test results to Der p extract before or after treatment in both the active and placebo groups. IgG4 levels significantly increased in the active group at 3 and 6 months and decreased at 12 months post-treatment.

As recommended by the World Allergy Organization, the minimal clinically relevant efficacy should be at least 20% higher than that in the placebo group. Despite the indicators and overall improvement rate being better in the active group than the placebo group, the effect of intratonsillar immunotherapy may dissipate over time. Therefore, further studies are needed.

ALLERGEN IMMUNOTHERAPY COMBINED WITH OMALIZUMAB

Omalizumab is a recombinant DNA-derived humanized monoclonal antibody that binds to IgE. Although omalizumab has currently been approved only for asthma and chronic spontaneous urticaria, studies have been carried out where AIT has been given in combination with omalizumab for AR, food allergy, and venom hypersensitivity. The first randomized, double-blind, placebo-controlled, trial was conducted by Kuehr et al. Combination therapy reduced the symptoms by 48%. Casale et al. investigated omalizumab pretreatment as an adjunct to rush IT with ragweed allergen. Those receiving combination therapy had lower symptom scores compared to monotherapy with AIT alone. The risk of anaphylaxis with SCIT was reduced by fivefold.

■ SUBCUTANEOUS IMMUNOTHERAPY WITH DUPILUMAB

Dupilumab is a monoclonal antibody that blocks the IL-4 receptor α. It not only regresses the polyps but also reduces type 2 serum biomarkers including total IgE. In this single-center, retrospective analysis, Dupilumab was administered in combination with SCIT. The nasal mucosal lining fluid (nMLF), serum samples, and clinical parameters were analyzed of patients suffering from AR and chronic rhinosinusitis with nasal polyps (CRSwNP) treated for 6 months with dupilumab. All patients were sensitized to at least one aeroallergen. After giving dupilumab treatment for 6 months, there was a significant decline in allergen-specific IgE levels, with some levels dropping below the detection limit. This reduction was more pronounced in nMLF than in serum. In some patients, there was also a decrease in both seasonal and perennial allergens. Additionally, total IgE levels decreased in both serum and nMLF. This reduction in IgE levels was accompanied by a significant improvement in allergic symptoms, as measured by a visual analog scale and the TNSS.

■ SUMMARY

As we are trying to understand the complex nature of the pathophysiology of AR, more research molecules are emerging. Multiple interacting, interdependent, and redundant pathways and molecular and cellular constituents are involved in the pathogenesis of AR. Every patient's response depends on many factors, such as genetics, epigenetics, and environment. A wider need for targeted therapies is the need and these new molecules are the future of AR treatment.

■ KEY POINTS

- Intranasal barrier molecules have shown benefits in seasonal AR.
- Setipiprant, roflumilast, resveratrol, LLLT, and antioxidants such as sodium pyruvate have shown results in reducing nasal inflammation.
- *CRISPR* gene editing technology is a breakthrough and has considerable implications for the new era of precision molecules.
- Allergen immunotherapy was developed based on the concept that if increasing quantities of the sensitizing allergen were given in specific doses at specific intervals, it leads to clinical tolerance. However, there was a risk with SCIT, and due to the longer duration of treatment adherence being poor, novel methods of AIT such as epicutaneous, intralymphatic, intratonsillar, and intradermal immunotherapy had to be developed.
- Monoclonal antibodies such as dupilumab have been restricted for severely affected patients as the cost of therapy by far exceeds the annual direct cost of medications.

SUGGESTED READING

1. Atipas K, Kanjanawasee D, Tantilipikorn P. Intradermal Allergen Immunotherapy for Allergic Rhinitis: Current Evidence. J Pers Med. 2022;12(8):1341.
2. Campion NJ, Doralt A, Lupinek C, Berger M, Poglitsch K, Brugger J, et al. Dupilumab reduces symptom burden in allergic rhinitis and suppresses allergen-specific IgE production. Allergy. 2023;78(6):1687-91.
3. Casale TB, Busse WW, Kline JN, Ballas ZK, Moss MH, Townley RG, et al. Omalizumab pretreatment decreases acute reactions after rush immunotherapy for ragweed-induced seasonal allergic rhinitis. J Allergy Clin Immunol. 2006;117(1):134-40.
4. Gupta N, Moitra S, Nagarajan S. Comprehensive textbook of allergy: Striking the right balance. New Delhi: Jaypee Brothers Medical Publishers (P) Ltd.; 2024.
5. Jung HJ, Chung YJ, Choi YS, Chung PS, Mo JH. Clinical Efficacy and Safety of Low-Level Laser Therapy in Patients with Perennial Allergic Rhinitis: a Randomized, Double-Blind, Placebo-Controlled Trial. J Clin Med. 2021;10(4):772.
6. Kuehr J, Brauburger J, Zielen S, Schauer U, Kamin W, Von Berg A, et al. Efficacy of combination treatment with anti-IgE plus specific immunotherapy in polysensitized children and adolescents with seasonal allergic rhinitis. J Allergy Clin Immunol. 2002;109(2):274-80.
7. Lee SR, Lee KL, Song SH, Joo MD, Lee SH, Kang JS, et al. Generation of Fel d 1 chain 2 genome-edited cats by CRISPR-Cas9 system. Sci Rep. 2024;14(1):4987.
8. Martin A, Lupfer C, Amen R. Sodium Pyruvate Nasal Spray Reduces the Severity of Nasal Inflammation and Congestion in Patients with Allergic Rhinitis. J Aerosol Med Pulm Drug Deliv. 2022;35(6):291-5.
9. Ojeda P, Piqué N, Alonso A, Delgado J, Feo F, Igea JM, et al. A topical microemulsion for the prevention of allergic rhinitis symptoms: results of a randomized, controlled, double-blind, parallel group, multicentre, multinational clinical trial (Nares study). Allergy Asthma Clin Immunol. 2013;9(1):32.
10. Popov TA, Emberlin J, Josling P, Seifalian A. In vitro and in vivo Evaluation of the Efficacy and Safety of Powder Hydroxypropylmethylcellulose as Nasal Mucosal Barrier. Med Devices (Auckl). 2020;13:107-13.
11. Ratner P, Andrews CP, Hampel FC, Martin B, Mohar DE, Bourrelly D, et al. Efficacy and safety of setipiprant in seasonal allergic rhinitis: results from Phase 2 and Phase 3 randomized, double-blind, placebo- and active-referenced studies. Allergy Asthma Clin Immunol. 2017;13:18.
12. Schmidt BM, Kusma M, Feuring M, Timmer WE, Neuhäuser M, Bethke T, et al. The phosphodiesterase 4 inhibitor roflumilast is effective in the treatment of allergic rhinitis. J Allergy Clin Immunol. 2001;108(4):530-6.
13. Senti G, Prinz Vavricka BM, Erdmann I, Diaz MI, Markus R, McCormack SJ, et al. Intralymphatic allergen administration renders specific immunotherapy faster and safer: a randomized controlled trial. Proc Natl Acad Sci U S A. 2008; 105(46):17908-12.
14. Senti G, von Moos S, Kündig TM. Epicutaneous Immunotherapy for Aeroallergen and Food Allergy. Curr Treat Options Allergy. 2013;1(1):68-78.
15. Stokes JR, Romero FA Jr, Allan RJ, Phillips PG, Hackman F, Misfeldt J, et al. The effects of an H3 receptor antagonist (PF-03654746) with fexofenadine on reducing allergic rhinitis symptoms. J Allergy Clin Immunol. 2012;129(2): 409-12, 412.e1-2.

16. Vogelberg C, Klimek L, Kruppert S, Becker S. Long-term effects of pollen allergoid tyrosine-adsorbed subcutaneous immunotherapy on allergic rhinitis and asthma. Clin Exp Allergy. 2024;54(4):253-64.
17. Zhang J, Yang X, Chen G, Hu J, He Y, Ma J, et al. Efficacy and safety of intratonsillar immunotherapy for allergic rhinitis: A randomized, double-blind, placebo-controlled clinical trial. Ann Allergy Asthma Immunol. 2024;132(3):346-354.e1.
18. Zhang W, Tang R, Ba G, Li M, Lin H. Anti-allergic and anti-inflammatory effects of resveratrol via inhibiting TXNIP-oxidative stress pathway in a mouse model of allergic rhinitis. World Allergy Organ J. 2020;13(10):100473.

Index

Page numbers followed by *b* refer to box, *f* refer to figure, *fc* refer to flowchart, and *t* refer to table.

A

Absolute eosinophil count 200
Acaricides 192
Acetylcholine 138
Acoustic rhinometry 83, 84, 86*f*, 89, 91*f*, 92, 96
    curve 87, 87*f*, 88*t*
        interpretation of 88
Adenoid 13
    evaluation of 70
    hypertrophy 20, 41, 45, 68*f*, 71, 71*f*, 72*f*
    X-ray for 70
Adhesive tape 95*f*
Adrenergic receptor agonist 142
Aeroallergens 33, 161
Air
    conditioner 7, 191*f*
    pollution 186
        traffic-related 36, 186
    pump 107*f*
    purifier systems 189
Air-filled cavities 16
Airways 71*f*, 101, 106*f*, 108*f*, 110
    pressure 108*f*
Allergenic components 126, 126*t*
Allergens 33, 116, 125, 126, 126*t*, 160, 162
    control 189
    exposures 185*t*
    immunotherapy 158, 162-164, 164*b*, 165, 183, 213, 216, 217
        contraindications of 159
        indications for 158
        safety of 163
    indoor 116
    interaction 173
    outdoor 116
Allergic asthma
    concomitant 168
    persistent 168
Allergic conjunctivitis 26, 45
    classification of 28
Allergic diseases 115, 187*f*, 196
    expression of 32
    systemic 46

Allergic disorders 197, 200, 204*t*
Allergic rhinitis 17, 19-21, 22*fc*, 30, 33*t*, 41, 60*f*, 83, 90, 91*f*, 94, 99, 104, 115, 131, 133*b*, 136, 137, 139, 141*t*, 146, 158, 162, 163, 167, 173-175, 196, 197, 200, 206, 209
    allergen-specific immunoprophylaxis of 189
    classification of 57*f*
    comorbidities 41
    diagnosis of 66
    etiology of 32
    intermittent 133
    local 21
    monotherapy for 156
    pathophysiology 32
    persistent 44, 133
    prevalence of 183
    seasonal 21, 61, 137, 139, 168, 190*f*
    structural analysis of 66
    treatment of 170, 198
Allergic spectrum, diseases of 46
Allergoids 164, 213
Allergy
    causation of 34
    prevention, three tiers of 184*f*
    protection 184
    tests 115
    treatment 189
Alprazolam 119
Aluminum hydroxide 164
Amiloride 54
Amitriptyline 54, 118
Amoxapine 118
Amruthaballi 119
Anaphylaxis 169
Angioedema 169
Angiotensin-converting enzyme 165
    inhibitors 54
Anticholinergics 138
    intranasal 141
Antihistamines 131, 133*b*, 135, 140, 154, 155, 155*t*
    first-generation 132

intranasal 119, 137
intraocular 119
oral 141, 146
recent use of 120
second-generation 133
third-generation 133
Antihypertensives 54
Anti-immunoglobulin E monoclonal
    antibody 166
Anxiety 197
Apathya 198
Arachis hypogaea 126
Arginases 106*f*
Arrhythmia 142
Asanas 203, 204
    practice 203
Ascomycetes 34
Aspergillus 34
Asthma 41, 42, 79, 133*b*, 136, 158, 159
    exacerbations 168
    severe 159
    worsening of 110
Asymmetric dimethylarginine 106*f*
    inhibits 105
Atopy, immunoprophylaxis of 189
Autoimmune 20
    disease 159
Autonomic nervous system 90
Ayurveda 196, 199
    medications 199
    nasya
        chikitsa 199
        procedure, demonstration of 199*f*
    physician 199
    treatment 197
Azelastine 118, 119, 137, 138, 155

B

Bambuterol 119
Baseline respiratory parameters diagnose
    asthmatics, measurement of 100
Basidiomycetes 34
Bat principle 84
Beclomethasone 147
Behavior therapies 206
Benralizumab 169
Benzodiazepines 119
Bepotastine 118
Beta-adrenergic blockers 54
Beta-blocker therapy 159
Bhunamanasana 204
Bilastine 136, 137

Biological
    drugs 170
    mechanism of action of 166*fc*
Blattella germanica 34, 126
Blomia tropicalis 160
Blood-brain barrier 132
Body
    circadian rhythm of 98
    mass index 111
Bone mineral density 150
Brain 210
Breastfeeding 187
Breathing
    normal 82
    practices 204
Brompheniramine 118
Bronchodilators
    inhaled 119
    oral plain 119
    parenteral 119
Bronchospasm 169
Budesonide 147

C

Calcium phosphate 164
Caldwell's view 70*f*
    digital 70
Candida 34
Canis lupus familiaris 126
Carbinoxamine 118
Carbon dioxide 36
Carcinoma 159
Cat allergen 35, 214
Cataract 152
    formation 150
Catecholamines 98
Cationic amino acid transport
    system 105, 106*f*
Cavity, oral 108*f*
Cells 38
    antigen-presenting 35, 215
Cellular response 38
Cellulose 119
Central compartment atopic disease 27
Central nervous system 63, 133, 134*f*
Cerebrospinal fluid leaks 20
Cetirizine 118, 136
Chemosis 45
Chest 62
Chlordiazepoxide 119
Chlorpheniramine 118, 132
Chlorpromazine 54, 119

Chromosomes 33
Chronic inflammatory disorder 41
Chronic obstructive pulmonary
    disease 109, 209
Ciclesonide 148
Cimetidine 119
Cinnarizine 118
Citalopram 119
Citrus unshiu powder 119
Clemastine 118
Climate change 186
Clobazam 119
Clonazepam 119
Clorazepate 119
Cockroach allergy 162, 192
Cognitive behavioral therapy 206
Computed tomography,
    contrast-enhanced 72
Congestion 89, 141, 143
Conical fibromuscular tube 12
Conjunctival allergen provocation test 122
Conjunctival diseases, allergic 28fc
Conjunctival irritation 51, 52
Conjunctivitis 41
    allergic 26, 45
    giant papillary 29
Coronavirus disease 2019 211
Corticosteroids 142, 151, 155, 155t
    inhaled 109, 112
    oral 109
    systemic 156
Cromoglycates 139
Cromolyn sodium 140
Cuticle 34
Cyclic guanosine monophosphate 106f
Cyclizine 118
Cyclooxygenase 214
Cyclosporine A 118
Cyproheptadine 118
Cystic fibrosis 27
Cytokines 167

D

Decongestants 141, 143, 154, 155t
    general adverse effects of 142
    oral 141
Dendritic cells 210
Dennie-Morgan lines 62f
Deoxyribonucleic acid methylation
    changes 33
Depression 197
Dermatitis, atopic 41, 46

Dermatographism, severe 120
Dermatophagoides
    farinae 160
    pteronyssinus 33, 160, 216
Desipramine 118
Desloratadine 118, 136
Deuteromycetes 34
Dexchlorpheniramine 118
Diazepam 119
Digital signal processors 191f
Dimenhydrinate 118
Dimethindene 118
Dimethylarginine, asymmetric 106f
Diphenhydramine 118, 132
Diurnal variation 53, 90
    calculation of 98
Dog allergen 35
Doshas 199
Doxepin 118
Drug 118, 119
    history 54
    interaction 151, 154
Dupilumab 168, 170, 217
Dust mite 160
Dyskinesia, primary ciliary 27

E

Ear 9f, 59
    anatomy 9, 18
    divisions 9f
    inner 10
    physiology 11, 18
Ebastine 118, 136, 137
Endoscopic sinus surgery 175, 177
Enzyme-linked immunosorbent assay 214
Eosinophil 112
    cationic protein 210
    interpretation of 112t
Ephedrine 141
Epigenetics 32
Epipharynx 13
Episodes, acute 198
Epistaxis 139, 150
Epithelial cells 210
Escitalopram 119
Estazolam 119
Ethmoid 7, 8, 77f, 90
    bilateral 73f
Etokimab 170
Euroglyphus maynei 160
Eustachian tube 10, 16f
    critical opening pressure of 18

Exercise 90
Exhaled nitric oxide 107
Expiratory flow rate 107f
   monitor 107f
   sensor 107f
External auditory canal 9
Eye 59
   itching 45
   redness 198
   watering 45
Eyeball, outer layer of 122

F

Face mask 95f
Famotidine 119
Felis domesticus 126
Femur, aseptic necrosis of 151
Fexofenadine 118, 135, 136, 211
Fibrosis, pulmonary 211
Fish oil supplements 187
Flunisolide 147
Fluorescence enzyme immunoassay 124
Fluoxetine 119
Fluphenazine 119
Fluticasone 155
   furoate 148, 155, 156
   propionate 148
Fluvoxamine 119
Food allergens 36
Forced expiratory volume 100
Formoterol 119
Fractional exhaled nitric oxide 105, 107f, 108f, 109-111
   interpretation 111t
   measurement system 107f
   use of 112
   values 111, 111t
Fresh air ventilator systems 190
Fungal spores 116

G

Gabapentin 54
Gallus gallus domesticus 126
Genes 33, 33t
   loci 32
Glaucoma 150
Glucocorticoids
   oral 151
   systemic 151
Granulocyte-macrophage colony-stimulating factor 132f

Granulomatosis 27
   eosinophilic 27
Guanosine triphosphate 106f

H

H1 blocker antihistamines 132
   adverse effects of 134, 134f
   first-generation
      long-action 118
      short-acting 118
   second-generation
      long-acting 118
      short-acting 118
Halitosis 198
Haridra khanda 199
Hay fever 190f
   symptoms 190f
Headache 142
Hearing, physiology of 12fc
High-efficiency particulate air filter unit 189
Histamine
   effects 211
   plasma levels of 98
Holt's proposal 189
House dust mite 33, 116, 126, 160
   allergens 160
   exposure 186
   sensitization 184
Human immunodeficiency virus 109
Humanized anti-immunoglobulin E monoclonal antibody 167
Humidity control machine 191, 191f
Hydralazine 54
Hydroxypropyl methylcellulose 209
Hydroxyzine 118
Hyperdense 75f
Hyperemia, conjunctival 45
Hyperresponsiveness, severe bronchial 110
Hypertension 142, 152
Hypertonic saline 142
Hypertrophy 68f
Hypopharynx 14
Hypotension 169

I

Ibuprofen 54
Imipramine 118
Immune prophylaxis, component-resolved 190f

Immunodeficiency 159
Immunoglobulin A 17, 27
Immunoglobulin E 17, 37, 63, 115, 132f, 166, 174, 190f
  desensitizing therapy for 158
  responses 209
Immunologic intervention, allergen-specific 190f
Immunoprophylaxis, allergen-specific 189, 190f
Immunotherapy 160, 161, 164
  allergen-specific 164, 186, 190f
  epicutaneous 215
  intradermal 215
  intralymphatic 214
  intratonsillar 215
  specific 159, 170
  use of 162
In vitro allergy tests 123
In vivo allergy tests 115
Infections 151
  fungal 74f, 75f, 77f
Inferior turbinate
  laser vaporization of 175
  reduction 174, 175
Inflammation 174
  allergic 38
  eosinophilic 104
Inflammatory cells, cytoplasm of 146
Infundibulum 5, 77f
Insects 116
Insomnia 142
Inspiratory peak nasal inspiratory flow 80
Interleukin 37, 166, 174f, 210
Interpreting allergy test 127
Intranasal corticosteroids 146, 147t, 149, 154, 155, 155t
  usage of 149f
Intranasal cromolyn 141
Itching 51

J

Jala neti 201, 202
  practice, demonstration of 203f

K

Kapalabhati 202
Kapha dosha dominant pratishaya 198
Keratoconjunctivitis, atopic 28
Ketotifen 118
Kriyas 201

L

Lacrimal
  apparatus 12
  fluid, pathway of 12fc
  gland 12
Lactation 147, 148
Langerhans cells 215
L-arginine 106f
  analogue 106f
Laryngopharyngeal physiology 15
Laryngopharynx 14
  anatomical relations of 15f
Larynx, critical opening pressure of 15, 18
Laser therapy, low-level 213, 214
Lebrikizumab 170
Leukocyte count 200
Leukotriene
  inhibitors 153t
  receptor antagonist 118, 152, 154, 155t
  synthesis 152
Levocabastine 137
Levocetirizine 118, 136
Levosalbutamol 119
Lipid microemulsion 210
Liposomes 164
Long-chain polyunsaturated fatty acid 187
Loratadine 118
Lorazepam 119
Lower airways
  functions 79, 83, 97
  protection of 7
  tests for 79
Lycopus lucidus 119
Lymph nodes, palpate neck for 60
Lymphoid tissue, nasal-associated 45

M

Machine, operating system of 191f
Magnetic resonance imaging 74, 76f, 77f
Major histocompatibility complex 37, 173
Malondialdehyde levels 210
Mammalian allergen, source of 214
Markatasana 204
Mask 80, 93
  placement of 81f
Mast cell 37
  stabilizers 139
Maxillary antrum 77f
Maxillary bones, palatine processes of 4
Maxillary sinusitis 73f-76f
Meclizine 118
Mental afflictions 197

Mepolizumab 169
Mepyramine 118
Mesoridazine 119
Messenger ribonucleic acid 149
Microcrystalline 209
    tyrosine 164
Microphone 85
Middle ear 11f
    cavity 16f
Mindfulness 205
Mini rhinoconjunctivitis quality of life questionnaire 216
Mizolastine 118
Mold 34, 126
Molecular-spreading process, evidence of 189
Molecules, generation of 211
Mometasone 148, 155
    furoate 156
Monitoring asthma symptoms 99
Monoclonal antibodies 168-170, 217
Monophosphoryl lipid A 164
Montelukast 118, 152, 153
    bilastine 155
    desloratadine 155
    fexofenadine 155
    levocetirizine 155
Mouth pressure 107f
Mucosa, atrophy of 142
Multicenter allergy study 190f
Mydriasis 142
Myopathies 151

N

Nasal
    adapters 86f
    air leaks 89
    airway 60f
        resistance, evaluation of 95
    allergen provocation test 122
    anatomy
        evaluation of 90
        examination of 90
    antihistamines 141
    bleed 142
    block 79
    cannula 95f
    cavity 4, 59, 60f, 77f, 84f, 108f
        X-ray for 69
    congestion 51, 141-143, 202, 211
        symptoms 212
    crease 58f
    cycle 7, 90, 94
    decongestants 141
    dysfunction 42
    endoscopy 67
    eosinophils 112
    filters 193
    irrigation 201
    irritation 142
    itch 141
    lavage fluid cytokine levels 210
    medication 199
    microemulsion, topical 210
    mucosa 67, 73f, 211
        inflammation of 112
        lining fluid 217
        structure 90
    obstruction 66, 82, 173, 174
    passage 66, 94
    patency 96t
    polyps 26, 26t, 61f, 174, 217
    provocation test 121
    pruritus 66
    reflexes 6, 7
    septum 3, 77f
    smear 112, 112t
    solution 140
    spray 142, 143, 150
    stuffiness 79
    symptoms, chronic 54t
    thudicum 67f
    tissue 210
    topical microemulsions 193
    turbinates, hypertrophy of 75f
    vestibule 4
    window 86f
Nasalis 3
Nasopharyngeal tonsil 13
Nasopharynx 13, 68f
    anatomical relations of 15f
Neck 60
    lateral soft tissue X-ray of 72f
Nedocromil 140
Neti pot 202f
Neurectomy 174
Neuropsychiatric disorders 152
Neurotransmitters, role of 39
Nitrative-oxidative stress 105, 106f
Nitric oxide 104, 108f, 109
    lung synthesis of 105
    metabolism 106f
    synthase 104, 106f
Nitrogen dioxide 36

Nonallergic rhinitis 20, 22
   pathophysiology of 19
Nonsteroidal anti-inflammatory drugs 54, 63
Nortriptyline 118
Nose 57
   anatomy of 3, 17, 91*f*
   external dimensions of 90
   floor of 66
   function of 17
   lateral wall of 4*f*
   physiology 6
   vestibule of 88
Nostril 155

O

Obesity 42
Obstructive sleep apnea 79
Olfaction 6
Olopatadine 118, 119, 137, 155
   nasal spray 138
Omalizumab 118, 166-168, 171, 216
   effect of 170
Oomycetes 34
Oral allergy syndrome 56
Orbital involvement 75
Oropharynx 14, 59
   anatomical relations of 15*f*
Osteocartilaginous framework 3
Osteoporosis 151
Ostiomeatal complex 27
Otitis media 29, 41, 46
Otoendoscopy 66
Otoscopy 69
Ovalbumin 210
Oxazepam 119
Oxymetazoline 142, 143, 155

P

Palatine tonsil 14
Panchakosha 201*f*
Pansinusitis 75*f*
Paranasal sinuses 7, 16
   anatomy 7
   overview 7*t*
   physiology of 9, 18
   X-ray for 69
Paroxetine 119
Pascolizumab 170
Pathya 198
Peak flow meter, parts of 98*f*

Peak nasal
   expiratory flow 80, 97
   inspiratory flow 79, 80, 82, 96
      application of 83
Penicillium 34
Perennial allergic rhinitis 21, 61, 137, 167, 168
Periplaneta americana 34
Perphenazine 119
Pharynx 12, 15*f*
   anatomical divisions of 13*f*
   cobblestone appearance of 62*f*
Pheniramine 118
Phenothiazines 119
Phenylephrine 141, 142
Phenylpropanolamine 141
Phosphodiesterase inhibitors 54, 212
Pitta dosha dominant pratishaya 198
Pollen 25, 126, 186
   allergen 161
   filter units 190
Polyangiitis 27
Polypoidal lesion 77*f*
Polyps
   large 75*f*
   nasal 26, 26*t*, 61*f*, 174, 217
      cavity for 59
Postcricoid region 15
Posterior pharyngeal wall 15
Postnasal drip 51, 52
Pranayama 205
Pranlukast 152, 153
Pratishaya 197
   prodromal symptoms of 197
Prazosin 54
Prebiotics 186
Pregnancy 120, 159
   period of 183
Probiotics 186, 192
Procerus muscle 3
Prochlorperazine 119
Proinflammatory cytokines, levels of 211
Promazine 119
Promethazine 118, 132
Prostaglandin 210, 212, 214
Protein pump inhibitors 119
Protriptyline 118
Provocation tests 121
Pseudoephedrine 141, 143
Psychiatric disorders, severe 159
Psychotropics 54
Pulmonary function test 133
Pyriform sinus 15

R

Radiofrequency
  ablation 175, 176
  coablation 175, 176
Raktaj pratishaya 198
Ranitidine 119
Reactive oxygen species 210
Reslizumab 169
Respiration 6
Respiratory mucous membrane 6
Respiratory system 79
Resveratrol 210
Rhinitis 19, 56, 63*fc*, 104, 110
  allergic 17, 19-21, 22*fc*, 30, 33*t*, 41, 60*f*, 83, 90, 91*f*, 94, 99, 104, 115, 131, 133*b*, 136, 137, 139, 141*t*, 146, 158, 162, 163, 167, 173-175, 196, 197, 200, 206, 209
    causes of 19, 20*b*
    chronic 19, 21*fc*
    classification 19
    clinical diagnosis of 51
    drug-induced 23
    gustatory 24
    hormonal 24
    idiopathic nonallergic 23
    infectious 19, 22
    medicamentosa 142
    nonallergic 20, 22
    noninfectious 19
    occupational 24
    pattern of 61*t*
Rhinoconjunctivitis, allergic 137, 165*fc*
Rhinomanometry 92, 94, 96, 101
  acoustic 85
  active anterior 95*f*
  anterior 92, 93, 94*f*
  four-phase 93
  posterior 93
Rhinometry 83
  acoustic 83, 84, 86*f*, 89, 91*f*, 92, 96
  machine 93
Rhinopathy, nonallergic 23
Rhinorrhea 51, 52, 131, 141
  anterior 66
  posterior 66
  watery 66
Rhinosinusitis 20, 24, 25, 41
  acute 25*fc*
    bacterial 25
  allergic fungal 27
  chronic 26, 26*t*, 27, 44, 110, 174, 217
  complications of 68
  eosinophilic chronic 27
  primary chronic 27*fc*
  recurrent acute 26
  secondary chronic 27*fc*
  viral 25
Rhizopus 34
Risperidone 54
Rodent allergen 36
Roflumilast 212

S

Salbutamol 119
Saline irrigation 149
Saliva 34
Salmeterol 119
Seasonal allergic rhinitis 21, 61, 137, 139, 168, 190*f*
  birch pollen-induced 167
Selective nasal tissue reduction 174
Selective norepinephrine reuptake inhibitors 119
Selective serotonin reuptake inhibitors 119
Senile rhinitis 23
Sensitization
  allergen-induced 174*f*
  phase 37*fc*
  profiles 116
Septal perforation 150
Septoplasty 175, 177
Septum 66
Sertraline 119
Setipiprant 212
Setu bandhasana 204
Shavasana 204
Sildenafil 54
Sinonasal squamous cell carcinomas 76
Sinuses 8*f*, 70*f*, 71*f*
  bilateral frontal 77*f*
  computed tomography of 74
  disease 68
  magnetic resonance imaging for 74
  mucosa, normal 67
Sinusitis 24, 44
Sinusoidal oscillography 95*f*
Sitopaladi churna 199
Skin 117, 118
  response 117
Skin prick test 45, 115, 117*f*, 118*t*, 120*f*, 158, 165
  contraindications of 120
  procedure 116

selection of antigens for 116
sensitivity of 117
specificity of 117
Sleep
   affecting quality of 131
   disorder 56
      breathing, detection of 96
   disturbances, identification of 94
   quality, assessment of 94
   wake cycle 98
Sneezing 51, 52, 66, 141
S-nitrosothiols 106f
Sodium pyruvate 211
Soluble guanylate cyclase 106f
Sonic tube 86f
Specific immunoglobulin E test 123
Sphenoid 7, 8, 77f
   sinusitis 77f
Spirometry 99, 100f
   role of 99
Spirulina 119
Steroids 98
   topical 118
Stress 197
Subcutaneous immunotherapy 158, 159, 160t, 161, 161t, 163, 165, 171, 188, 214, 217
Sublingual immunotherapy 158, 159, 161, 161t, 163, 165, 188
Sublingual vaccinations 162
Submucosal resection 175, 176
Superoxide dismutase level 210
Surgery, indications for 174
Sutra neti 202
   catheter 203f
   practice, demonstration of 204f
Synechiae formation 176

T

Tachycardia 142
Tadalafil 54
Temazepam 119
Terbutaline 119
Tezepelumab 170
Theophylline 118
Therapeutic interventions, evaluation of 90
Thiol groups 106f
Thioridazine 119
Thymic stromal lipoprotein 170
Thyroid gland 60

Tonsils 14
   physiological role of 14
Total immunoglobulin E test 123
Total nasal symptom score 191, 216
Toxicity 135
Tralokinumab 170
Tranquilizers 119
Transient nasal dryness 139
Triamcinolone acetonide 147, 156
Triazolam 119
Tricyclic antidepressants 118
Tridosha balance 197
Trifluoperazine 119
Triflupromazine 119
Trimipramine 118
Tube system 85
Tulasi 119
Tumors 59
Tympanic membrane 59

U

Upper airway 17, 79
   critical opening pressure of 15
   defensive mechanisms of 17t
   normal defense mechanisms of 16
   physiology 3
   role of 17
   tests for 79
Urticaria 167, 169
Ustrasana 204

V

Vardenafil 54
Vasa avaleha 199
Vata dosha dominant pratishaya 198
Vernal keratoconjunctivitis 28
   limbal 28
   mixed 28
   palpebral 28
Vertebrae, anatomical divisions of 13f
Vestibular system 11
Vidian neurectomy 175, 178
Vienna speculum 67f
Vijñānamaya kosha 200
Vipassana 205
Vitamin 187

W

Waters view, digital 70, 71
World Allergy Organization 216

X

Xylometazoline 142-144

Y

Yoga 200, 205, 206
    postures 203
    practices 204*t*

Yogic breathing 205
Yogic cleansing techniques 201
Youlten's nasal peak flow meter 80, 81*f*

Z

Zafirlukast 118, 152, 153
Zileuton 152, 153
Zygomycetes 34

EU GSPR Authorised Reprsentative
Logos Europe, 9 rue Nicolas Poussin
1700, La Rochelle, France
Phone: +33 (0) 6 67 93 73 78
E-mail: contact@logoseurope.eu

www.ingramcontent.com/pod-product-compliance
Ingram Content Group UK Ltd.
Pitfield, Milton Keynes, MK11 3LW, UK
UKHW051846210426
5322IPUK00019B/277